UNDERSTANDING DISEASE

A Health Practitioner's Handbook

John Ball

Index compiled by
Francesca Garwood-Gowers

SAFFRON WALDEN
THE C.W. DANIEL COMPANY LIMITED

First published in Great Britain
by Blackdown Publications
This revised and updated edition
published in Great Britain by
The C.W. Daniel Company Limited
1 Church Path, Saffron Walden, Essex, England.

© John Ball 1990

ISBN 0 85207 229 5

Designed by Peter Dolton.

Design and Production in association
with Book Production Consultants, Cambridge, England.

Typeset by Anglia Photoset, Colchester
Printed and bound by The Bath Press, Avon.

Contents

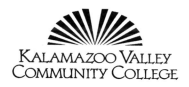

FOREWORD

Culled from his training and experience in orthodox practice (Dr Ball was a GP from 1970 81), and also from teaching at various schools and colleges of complementary medicine, the author has written a book which addresses the former from the standpoint of the requirements of the latter. Its primary purpose is to describe pathological processes in the language of orthodoxy while offering explanations in simple and clarifying terms. It is a book of immense utility. Those who have come to health care through a route other than medical school will appreciate the value of a systematic analysis of disease, and through familiarity with the language of pathology be able to communicate with their medical colleagues. There is no doubt in my mind that there are only gains to be made out of bringing these two apparently disparate approaches into communion. The process is, I believe, similar to any 'marriage of opposites', a necessary step in the direction of wholeness and maturity.

The medical doctor, traditionally observing the tenets of his Hippocratic Oath, is not permitted to divulge medical knowledge. The times are changing in this respect as well as in respect of acknowledging the limitations of this system of medicine. The treatment which it offers is often suppressive, usually productive of iatrogenic side-effects and leads to various long term though often unacknowledged consequences.

The premise upon which most forms of complementary medicine stand is that the symptoms are the language by which the diseased organism finds expression. They are the outward evidence of the internal disorder, providing the healer/physician with a true guide, like Dante's Virgil, a lead into the hidden interior wherein the disturbance is centered. Furthermore, the symptoms are understood to represent the best possible adaptation which the organism can muster in order to save itself from a deeper, more permanent and more destructive form of disturbance. From this point of view it is self evident that any form of treatment which suppresses the symptoms will inevitably lead to the eventual intensification of the suffering.

However, this conclusion is usually not drawn because it is assumed that the disease is an entity in itself, a unique syndrome of symptoms, independent of the sufferer and therefore dealt with as if it were an enemy – attacked and destroyed. This view closes the mind to further possibilities, because once the symptoms have been extinguished it is deemed *a priori* that the disease has been vanquished. Another reason for the lack of a true interpretation of the disease is due to the habit of compartmentalising the information which is received from the patient. Spirit, emotions, mind and body are each treated as though separate; even the physical body is subdivided and specialists consulted whose role is to examine, diagnose and eventually treat the parts.

Practitioners of complementary medicine tend to emphasise a synthetic and embracing philosophy of healing; it is because of this bias that they need to pay particular attention to the paradigm of Western medicine, itself an outcome of the reductionist and casual model of reality. This model is powerful because the manipulation of concepts leads to mastery of matter. However, mind may be divorced from feeling in the interest of expediency. This unilateral view is responsible for much mischief, for feeling associates while reason isolates. Suffering is a common concomitant of civilisation; its alleviation may be sought through an awareness of soul processes and the reconnection to the spiritual heart, the feeling centre of our life's purpose. Having made this statement it must nonetheless be born in mind that the great insights of science may be used for the benefit of man, no less in the field of healing. Medical science, with its store of observation, the accumulated evidence of centuries of recording and correlation contains testimony to both the miracle of life and the tragedy of disease. It is a description of the physical field within which we find ourselves. Unlike the treatment which is offered on the basis of dubious premises, the description of the body and the pathology it is heir to cannot be refuted.

Misha Norland.

PREFACE

*T*his book has evolved from several years of lecturing and discussing the often controversial topic of disease with homoeopaths, osteopaths, herbalists, acupuncturists and other healing professionals. Each of these disciplines has its own map of the human mind and body, and the ills which befall them, and most recognise that to try to construct a single all-encompassing model describing the human condition is to attempt the impossible, so an understanding of different viewpoints is needed for the complete picture. Indeed the resurgence of interest in alternative methods of pursuing health is largely due to the emphasis which science has placed on disease processes, to the point where the patient and his or her suffering has been supplanted.

Any realistic approach to illness must include an objective appraisal of the dysfunction of the body (pathology), an understanding of how the patient sees the problem (empathy) and a philosophy of diagnosis and treatment which may involve a wide range of perspectives and skills. What follows is an attempt to walk a tightrope between knowledge and understanding, so that the science of pathology and all its clinical manifestations becomes comprehensible without the dubious necessity of surrounding oneself with a fortification of information for its own sake, which is as able to erect barriers as destroy them. Hence the book is hopefully not a catalogue of diseases but an appraisal of the disorders likely to be seen in the average working life of a practitioner. Rare diseases hold the same sort of fascination for medical authors as rare birds do for birdwatchers and most medical texts give a disproportionate amount of consideration to once-in-a-lifetime problems. This may mean that some readers will feel short-changed by the absence of parathyroid disorders for example, but the line has to be drawn somewhere, and those conditions affecting less than 1 in 20,000 of the population have been ignored or only mentioned in passing. If the core of medical science is understood the patient with a rare disease can be pursued in standard texts.

An understanding of the structure and function of the human body has been assumed, there is not enough space to include anatomy and physiology, nor more than a brief description of orthodox treatment, although the drugs which are in common use today and their main side effects have been included as these are becoming questioned more by an increasingly sophisticated public. Medical terminology has been used where relevant, not because it is strictly necessary but rather because without a minimal understanding of the terms a student is unable to refer elsewhere nor a practitioner to explain the jargon to patients. As the majority of words are of Greek or Latin origin, the translation is given for clarity and interest and a glossary of terms appended at the back. This includes a number of words which are not in common usage today but appear in some of the classic texts of homoeopathy, and are so labelled.

Textbooks of medical science make depressing reading for those susceptible to suggestion, and many students may imagine themselves to be harbouring all manner of ills as they turn these pages. All I can say to them is that it probably isn't what you think and you probably won't get what you imagine!

My thanks are due especially to my friends Misha Norland and Tim Fox who have made many helpful suggestions about the contents, and to Donald, my father, who has ironed out many of the hiccoughs in the course of the book. Also to Dr Keith Ball for his pertinent comments on the chapters on the heart and vessels. Most of all to my family for their long-standing support and tolerance of my wraith-like disappearances for many hours on end.

CHAPTER ONE

HEALTH
PATHOLOGY AND
DISEASE

*T*he prevailing attitude of the majority of people today is the Cartesian one, that the world in general and the body in particular are the sum of their parts and can be dissected, analysed and adjusted to perform better. Orthodox medicine in fact looks on the body as a machine, and this is both its success and its failure. The failure of orthodoxy is its apparent inability to distinguish between the body and the person, and in making the assumption that they are identical. This is the inevitable consequence of the convergent, analytical approach based on specialisation, where increasing technology allows us to focus on ever smaller details of the 'machine' at the expense of the 'owner'. The success of orthodoxy lies in its refusal to be distracted from measurement, so that it has developed refined and logical techniques for describing, categorising, diagnosing and in some cases treating disease.

We are now moving, it seems, into a post-Cartesian era which can encompass other models of the body. The reason for the move appears to be two-fold, firstly the realisation by science itself that matter is relative, and secondly the willingness to embrace other belief systems as disillusionment with materialism increases – more and more of the same does not appear to be the solution. It is becoming apparent that the only way forward is to examine the whole ecological framework within which a 'disease' prospers and find ways of adjusting that environment so that the condition simply evaporates with the course of time. Indeed the model we are left with is that of the body as a continually changing process kept in dynamic equilibrium by its own internal gyroscopes. In short we are back to the Taoist philosophy of the 4th century BC.

It may be that patients understand this intuitively when they turn away from the academic citadels and seek out 'alternative' medicine. It may be that more and more practitioners sense this as they opt for alternative or complementary methods of healing, but whatever is the case it seems that what Werbach calls 'Third Line Medicine' is here to stay, and we are left finally with the realisation that a single model cannot encompass the huge intricacies of the human being and that circumstances alone can dictate our methods. This is not to say that there will be no need for the doctrine of specific causes, that would be to throw the baby out with the bathwater, but persistence with a single conceptual approach is likely to become less useful with time.

HEALTH

Although most of this book is concerned with diseases, we should perhaps start by looking at what constitutes health. This is not easy to define as everyone has their own concept of an ideal body with no physical, emotional or mental discomfort and a pervading sense of well-being and fitness. In purely physical terms health is a stable internal environment maintained in the face of external changes to which we have learned to adapt in the course of evolution. That is not to say that the adaptive process is always comfortable, in fact it is this very discomfort which we call 'suffering', but that is not the same as illness. What one individual will take in his or her stride may cause another great suffering, for one of the greatest barriers to health is not so much the illness itself but the emotional reaction to it. It is precisely because we have come to assume that science can provide a cure for every situation that we are now in a state of suffering, because our mind is so full of unfulfilled expectations.

The chronic effects of stress, pollution, faulty diet or unhappiness are subtle and do not begin to make themselves felt until the chain breaks at its weakest link and pathology shows itself in one form or another. Just to look at this pathology in isolation is to examine a single slice of a continuum of events, and it is important to realise that the same stimulus has been affecting other aspects of the body which may only later fail. Therefore to try and reverse that particular disclosure of the body without looking beyond is of limited benefit, although it may be worth doing.

It is certainly quite often the case that the physical aspects of disease, i.e. the pathology, can be influenced in some way by the scientific approach, but in most cases the physical manifestation is only the final expression of a process which has been continuing for a long time. What we have come to consider in the post-Cartesian era are the events which lead up to that change, and these events are usually in the realm of a different model.

THE ERA OF TOLERANCE

If pathology is the final expression of a provocation then we should perhaps be spending more time looking at the events leading up to the disease, rather than examining the disease itself. This may seem obvious and much has been written about the way in which our National Health Service has become a National Disease Service (Brian Inglis: The Diseases of Civilisation), but one of the main reasons why scant attention has been paid to prevention is because it is neither easily measurable nor very predictable.

If we look at the era which precedes the outbreak of pathology, the duration when external stimuli are apparently tolerated with impunity, we see no visible reaction, no measurable consequences. All that can be measured are the stimuli themselves, and as the Cartesian approach is to discard what cannot be quantified any idea that the body could be influenced by a self regulating 'tendency' within itself is also discarded as mere speculation. As is the possibility that as well as being disrupted by events the 'tendency' (for want of a better word) may fluctuate of its own accord and even be amenable to treatment.

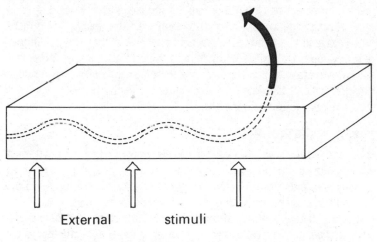

FIGURE 1.1   *The era of tolerance and the emergence of pathology*

To translate this into a three dimensional model as in Fig. 1.1 the Cartesian view will be from above, in which case nothing will appear to happen until the sudden emergence of a pathological state from below, and subsequent bodily changes. The direction and rate of change together constitute the shape which the pathology and therefore the disease takes, and this change can be opposed by a variety of methods, principally drugs and surgery.

Most complementary practitioners, however, view events in the model from the side, and therefore see something rather different. They must, of course, formulate some concept to explain what occurs in the 'era of tolerance' before the emergency of symptoms, and a wide variety of names have been given by various cultures from the Classical times onwards. These include Ch'i, the vital force, prana, the subtle body, and even the aura, and while there are those who would dispute the similarity between these terms, most of these disputes have more to do with the methods used to influence the direction of this 'force' than with the force itself.

Because the era of tolerance has not so far proved amenable to methods of objective study (Kirlian photography may be an exception to this), it has largely been dismissed as fanciful by scientists. And because any changes which take place are subjective they are generally felt by someone who is in a relatively undistracted state. This crucial fact leads to the curious and rather amusing situation that those who are distracted by seeking for objective evidence do not, by and large, experience their own inner feelings due to their very distraction with the search, while those who engage in such meditative practices as enable them to catch glimpses of it develop a fascination which tempts them to abandon measurement and even spurn it as unnecessary. It is these disparate views of the same situation which has created the two camps of health practice today, with their tendency to mutual repulsion.

EXPRESSIONS OF PATHOLOGY

When we use the word 'disease' we usually think of a recurring pattern of change found in certain people, often those of a similar age and sex, which is manifested either as subjective symptoms or as objective changes in the body. It mostly happens that the symptoms occur first – as pains, weakness, itching, tremor, disorientation, faintness etc, and only much later, if at all, do detectable changes happen to the body. Pathology is the name given to the study of changes in the tissues which result from some form of inadequacy of adaptation, and it is this study which forms the cornerstone of orthodox medicine.

The reasons why our adaptive mechanism fails may be inherent in our make up, or due to overwhelming challenge by some stimulus or another, and these types of failure account for the varieties of congenital and acute diseases. The majority of chronic illness is more complex than this, however, and is a combination of predisposition, inadequate defence and repeatedly maintained challenges in the form of nutrition, radiation etc. Faced with this the body has a variety of standard ways of expressing its discomfort, and these constitute the main varieties of pathology outlined below.

The experience of patients subjected to these forms of pathology will differ to some extent depending on the organs involved, the rapidity of onset and even their age, and it is these differences which account for the bewildering varieties of symptoms in any disease. In general the law of probability applies, in that the unusual symptoms of common conditions are far more likely to occur than the common manifestations of rare diseases. As far as diagnosis is concerned it is important to be able to work backwards as well, and use symptoms as a way of excluding or suggesting possible underlying pathology, and to bear in mind that the commonest reason for missing a diagnosis is because the possibility never crossed your mind. In this connection it is important to ask oneself what likely pathology could be encountered in a person of this age and sex and then ask specific questions at some point to unearth the necessary information.

INFLAMMATION

The standard response of the body to sudden challenge from heat, light, radiation, chemicals and micro-organisms is inflammation. This is characterised by the four classical symptoms of *pain, heat, swelling* and *redness.* When inflammation occurs there is a reaction in the local blood vessels, and this takes the form of dilation (causing redness and heat), followed by an increase in their permeability (causing the pain and swelling). This enables the phagocytes, those white cells responsible for engulfing foreign bodies, to migrate through the wall into the tissues, as well as the plasma proteins with their antibodies and clotting factors. The way in which the inflammatory reaction is quickly brought about is by the liberation of *histamine* and other chemicals, especially from the mast cells but also from others. Following this the reaction may quickly subside with minimal pain felt as itching (as in nettle stings), or be continued indefinitely as chronic inflammation by a group of chemicals first discovered in the prostate gland and therefore known as the *prostaglandins.*

Inflammation of one kind or another is seen in the majority of acute diseases, and swift resolution usually follows. If the inflammatory response is inadequate a much more prolonged situation may occur, as may be observed in such conditions as TB, syphilis, rheumatoid arthritis and Crohn's disease. The normal phagocytes of the blood, the polymorphs, are unable to do the job and hand it over to rather more specialised cells, the macrophages (lit. 'big eaters') which are modified monocytes that have left the blood stream and settled down to a long life in the tissues. There they can engulf very large particiles but in doing so produce large quantities of fibrous tissue which swells up to look like a tumour, so these swellings were given the name *granuloma* by the early pathologists and are the

5

charactistic feature of many chronic diseases.

The way in which the inflammatory response manifests and resolves is reflected in the symptoms of many diseases, particularly those classified as infections. In some there is complete and rapid resolution and such conditions as mumps and measles therefore run short and predictable courses. In others there may be areas of suppuration where the tissues break down and result in abscesses (collections of pus), ulcers and later scarring. Sometimes the organisms penetrate the containing tissues and invade the lymphatic or blood vessels to cause septicaemia and profound toxaemia (blood poisoning). In general the more specialised a tissue is the less it is able to regenerate after being inflamed, so that connective tissue such as bone will usually heal successfully but such tissues as nerves, kidney and muscle will be unable to re-grow, and non-functioning scar tissue will replace it.

TUMOURS

In most people's minds the word 'tumour' is synonymous with cancer, and this is a grave error in thinking, for the literal meaning is simply 'swelling'. Since we are composed of somewhere in the region of three trillion cells, and each of those cells has the ability to divide about 50 times in the course of our lifetime before the process grinds to a halt, it is highly likely that this process of division, or mitosis as it is called, may under certain circumstances become distorted to a greater or lesser extent. As a rule any abnormal cells will be eradicated by the immune system as if they were foreign to the body (see chapter 3), but if the changes are minimal then they can be overlooked and allowed to remain, though the changes incurred may be detectable under the microscope.

Two terms are applied to such minimal changes. The first is *metaplasia* (literally 'altered form'), which refers to a reversible change that is seen in a fairly complex cell whereby it reverts to a more simple state, such as is seen in the glandular epithelium of the cervix or the mucous membrane of the respiratory tract. This change is generally brought about by a continued stimulus which may be either chemical or inflammatory, and is the first indication that something is amiss. If the change proceeds to alteration in the size and shape of the cell as well, the the term *dysplasia* is used and this change is less likely to return to normal. Understandably, both types of altered growth are the result of many possible causes, the more obvious chemical ones being termed 'carcinogens' because of their long term consequences, and if these changes are untreated they become progressively abnormal culminating in a total escape from control. Since metaplasia and dysplasia are symptomless, this premalignant state can only be detected by some form of screening procedure involving examination of the tissue microscopically, and this is only worthwhile when the likelihood of preventing disease is fairly high.

Once total escape from control has occurred, *neoplasia* or 'new growth' is said to have happened and the coded instructions which the genes relay to the new cells become corrupted, leaving the cell to continue dividing but with no control over when to stop or how to differentiate into specialised tissue. If the former alone occurs then the neoplasia is said to be benign and the new cells may push aside their neighbours and cause symptoms due to pressure, but will not invade or infiltrate other tissues nor *metastasise* (spread by blood and lymph channels) to distant sites. Moreover the plethora of new cells will look very similar to their parents and closely resemble the tissue of origin.

But neoplasia is not always benign and if the cells are sufficiently damaged then the offspring will revert to primitive forms which do not differentiate into their specialised tissues and are thus said to be *undifferentiated* to a greater or lesser degree. In general the less differentiated a neoplasm is, the greater its degree of malignancy and vice versa. We can see then that the difference between a well differentiated malignant tumour and a benign tumour may be very slight and barely discernible under the microscope except by an experienced pathologist, yet this is of great significance when the question of prognosis and possible surgery arises.

Tumours are labelled according to their tissue of origin, and this may be epithelial tissue (mucus membrane or skin), glandular or connective tissue of one kind or another. Benign epithelial tumours look like smooth warts and may even have a small stalk so are termed *papillomas* (L. papilla = nipple). Because the epithelial surfaces of the body are most likely to come into contact with carcinogens many of the malignant tumours arise here and are known as *carcinomas* (Gr. carcinos = crab), and are usually prefixed by their tissue type, e.g. 'squamous cell carcinoma of bronchus', 'transitional cell carcinoma of bladder'.

Benign glandular tumours tend to arise in endocrine glands where they may lead to some of the malfunctions described in chapter 16 on hormonal disorders, and they are termed *adenomas* to distinguish them from the malignant *adenocarcinomas* (of which the commonest example is the breast). Connective tissue tumours which arise in fat, muscle, cartilage etc are common and almost always benign – for instance fibroids which are seen in the smooth muscle of the uterus, lipomas which may appear as soft fatty lumps under the skin. They are generally given the name of the tissue in which they arise with the suffix *-oma*, such as

7

fibroma, chondroma, osteoma. However on the few occasions where the connective tissues do produce malignant tumours, they are among the most malignant known and tend to arise in younger people. They are given the suffix -*sarcoma*, e.g. osteosarcoma, fibrosarcoma etc., after the Greek word 'sarx' meaning 'flesh'.

TABLE 1.1 The incidence of cancer in the UK	
Lung & Bronchus	31%
Breast	11%
Stomach	9%
Colon	9%
Lymph glands & Marrow	7%
Rectum	5%
Pancreas	5%
Prostate	5%
Bladder	4%
Oesophagus	3%
Ovary	2%
Leukaemia	2%
Cervix	2%

DEGENERATION

However much care we take of our bodies it is unfortunately a fact that they start to degenerate at a certain stage and although we can slow this process up we cannot reverse it to any great extent. This deterioration, which we know as ageing, starts at around 30–40 and is nature's way of ensuring that a large percentage of a single species does not continue to exist beyond reproductive age as this reduces the possibilities for the more vigorous members. Fortunately human society has been able to arrange things so that accumulated experience continues to dominate where physical prowess long since left the stage, but in this respect we are unusual in the animal kingdom, and experience only compensates as long as the underlying problems remain the same which is why new technology will always be the domain of youth.

It is rather ironic that degeneration often takes place most rapidly in those on whom the environment appears to lay least stress, and this is largely a modern phenomenon. A diet so rich in refined carbohydrate and saturated fat, coupled with little need to use the calories, has resulted in new forms of nutritional pathology such as diabetes and atheroma to replace those of rickets and 'chlorosis' as iron deficiency was once termed.

Overnutrition coupled with lack of exercise creates a net surplus in calories which the body preserves as fat rather than allowing it to go to waste. It does this both by increasing the number of adipose cells in the body and by increasing the amount of fat stored in each. The number of fat cells which a body contains is determined by the degree of nutrition in the first year of postnatal life, so that overfeeding during this period may as much as double the number of fat cells in the body and the tendency to corpulence will be permanent. This largely accounts for the extreme degree of obesity in some individuals, which no amount of dieting seems to resolve, as well as the tendency of some people to remain thin under all conditions.

Although each cell in the body is potentially immortal, in practice this never happens and cellular integrity collapses on average within a year, depending on just how successfully homeostasis is maintained. Once our body arrives at a point where it is composed of cells which are no longer actively dividing but can only deteriorate, the accumulated excesses will then exert rapid changes on a variety of organs and lead eventually to overt pathology, and this begins somewhere around late middle age. It is arguable exactly how degeneration and ageing come about, it may be because the blood supply becomes defective and the necessary oxygen and nutrients are not forthcoming, or it may be that accumulated toxins and chemicals build up and damage the delicate cells.

It is at this point that the osmotic pressure of the surrounding fluid will overwhelm the delicate pumping mechanism of the cell which will flood with water and swell. It is here that the accumulated fatty deposits in the walls of the vessels will obstruct the passage of blood and oxygen and lead to anoxia of the tissues. And it is now that our previously supple cartilage will become fixed with deposits of calcium salts in a vain attempt to strengthen weakening fibres. But ultimately we must all succumb to the failure of whichever organ we have, knowingly or unknowingly, abused the most, and by doing so begun the unravelling of the web which knitted together sustains our life.

CHAPTER TWO

ALLERGY: DISORDERS OF ECOLOGY

*N*ature has no interest in the survival of the human race. At least, no more so than any of the other species. She functions as the great balancer, a sort of free economy where different groups ebb and flow according to conditions. For millennia this is how life functioned and harmony reigned, until humans identified themselves as the most important of all the species, which must have been around the time when we started breeding animals for food, instead of hunting them and being hunted on equal terms. It still took a number of centuries for us to develop tools of sufficient destructive power to upset the balance of nature, but finally by the mid 20th century the stage was set. Pesticides and fertilizers ensured sufficient food, antibiotics and hygiene a longer life and the population exploded, leaving a trail of ecological damage which may take an equally long time to repair itself. In the late 20th century we are hopefully beginning to reverse the damage done not only to the environment but to ourselves as well. Great interest has arisen particularly in the fields of immunology and allergic disorders, and in the way in which our bodies react to pollution of all types. The name for this new approach is *clinical ecology*.

THE IMMUNE SYSTEM
Our natural ability to withstand outside interference from micro-organisms is assisted by several defence mechanisms (defensive from our point of view at any rate), and the chief of these is the immune system. Under normal circumstances, when an organism or other foreign protein is found in the body it is immediately 'arrested' and taken to the local lymph node, where certain cells known as *B lymphocytes* set to work and in a few days produce an identical progeny or 'clone' of plasma cells which in turn produce proteins called *antibodies*. These antibodies are specially fashioned so that they key into the protein coat of the invader, which is termed an *antigen* as it generates antibodies. This type of 'lock and key' configuration is together known as an 'immune complex', and renders the organism harmless until it can be removed by phagocytes. In case there are more organisms on the way, many more antibody 'keys' are made and

stored as *immunoglobulins* in the body, so that we are a warehouse of different types of antibody stored in readiness.

This, of course, is the basis for most types of immunisation. Some organisms like tetanus and scarlet fever try to beat the system by secreting powerful poisons called toxins which damage the host, but lymphocytes can produce antibodies against these proteins too in the form of antitoxins. Because most of these antibodies are stored in the blood they are termed *humoral antibodies* to distinguish them from other, *cell-mediated*, antibodies which are located in the cells of the tissues.

There is a possible snag, however, which is that the B lymphocytes must be careful not to make antibodies against parts of their own body, which they have to recognise. This is done by having a pair of 'educated' *T lymphocytes* supervising each B lymphocyte and either helping it or suppressing it, according to whether or not they recognise the protein. They are called T lymphocytes incidentally because they receive their 'education' at an early age in the thymus gland. If the T lymphocytes are damaged or make a wrong decision then either no antibody gets made and immunodeficiency results, or antibodies against the body's own tissues are formed and what is called an autoimmune disease may occur.

T lymphocytes also have another role to play, and as well as monitoring the activity of B lymphocytes they also produce a series of antibodies which do not circulate as immune complex in the blood stream but instead police the tissues as cell-mediated immunity. Their responsibility is to reject larger entities such as the large bacteria, fungi, cancerous cells and transplanted tissues, and because they take rather longer to act their reactions are known as *delayed hypersensitivity reactions*. A typical example of one of these is the Mantoux test for TB which takes several days to exhibit.

The earliest studies of the immune system were largely related to immunisation and vaccines, and it was only later that attention was switched to the phenomenon of allergy (Gr=other work) and hypersensitivity. This was something of a puzzle to investigators who had assumed that immune reactions could only benefit the host, but it seems that the system has evolved to over- rather than under-react and this is simply the price we have to pay for our defence. Indeed it is arguable that these reactions are always inappropriate, for they may be telling us that our body is uncomfortable with the way in which it is being treated.

ALLERGY

To understand this we need first to take a closer look at the immunoglobulins, those 'keys' made by the B lymphocytes. These come in five slightly different varieties or classes, each with a specific role to play, and each is therefore given a distinguishing letter. Starting with the most abundant the letters are G, A, M, D and E, so because they are all immunoglobulins these are abbreviated to IgG, IgA, IgM, IgD and IgE.

IgG forms the majority and circulates throughout the blood and tissues, even crossing the placenta. Along with IgM it forms the majority of the immune-complexes mentioned earlier. IgA is located especially in the secretions of the gut and has a role to play in hypersensitivity to foods (see next section). IgD does not appear to have been found a very significant role as yet, but it is IgE, the antibody which is least abundant, that causes the most allergic problems.

It has long been known that certain individuals react in a specific but unpleasant way each time they come into contact with certain substances – usually house dust, animal fur or pollen in the air – and so they were named *atopic* which means literally 'out of place'. Atopy runs in families and manifests clinically as asthma, hay fever and eczema, and it is known that atopic children have up to six times the normal amounts of IgE, located in the skin and mucus membranes. The actual cells in which IgE is found are called *mast cells*, and when stimulated they release large quantities of histamine and other similar chemicals very rapidly, which cause smooth muscle to contract and vessels to leak fluid in large quantities – the very symptoms of asthma and hay fever. This is one of the commonest and most studied of the hypersensitivity reactions, and is sometimes classified as *type 1 hypersensitivity.*

In a few individuals the type 1 hypersensitivity is widespread and of a more dramatic nature, and they may suffer a sudden severe reaction after an injection of a foreign substance such as penicillin or an immunisation of some kind. Shortly afterwards they are liable to collapse and have difficulty breathing, with a sudden drop in blood pressure, a condition called *anaphylaxis* or anaphylactic shock (Gr. = to ambush).

It was noticed that the condition of *urticaria*, also called *hives* or *nettlerash*, happens occasionally after eating certain foods such as shellfish, strawberries, eggs or even the chemicals present in them as dyes or preservatives. This condition must operate through IgE as the reaction is so swift, often within half an hour or so, and produces the typical evidence of a histamine reaction with swelling, itching etc. Sometimes the reaction is general and all the tissues swell, most noticeably those of the eyelids, throat and lips, all of which contain tissues which are loosely bound – *angio-oedema*. Here, then, is a food allergy with all the ingredients for anaphylaxis present, and it is possible that this could be the explanation for some cases of 'cot death' in young babies. But in this case

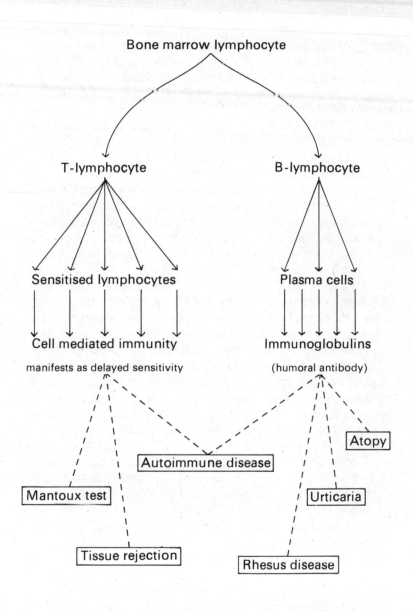

FIGURE 2.1   *The mechanism and possible consequences of immunity*

what is the means of introduction of the allergen, as no inoculation is evident? There is good evidence that cot death occurs around the time of weaning when new foods are being introduced and that it is more common in non breast fed babies. It was considered that allergy to cow's milk could be a cause, and this has lead to the speculation that food is more involved in the whole spectrum of illness than had been previously thought.

FOOD INTOLERANCE

The reactions to some foods such as have just been described are clear-cut and dramatic, even though the exact ingredient which triggers the reaction is not always obvious. In practice, however, many patients seek help for symptoms which do not fit clearly into a textbook picture of disease – symptoms like headache, catarrh, diarrhoea, distension, depression and a host of others. Or if they do fit into a disease category, it is one for which no clearcut cause has emerged, such as ulcerative colitis or rheumatoid arthritis, and some of these patients, though by no means all, respond dramatically to what is called an elimination diet.

What is the mechanism by which some foods appear to lead to these adverse reactions and why are they 'masked', i.e. delayed? This question is at the core of the controversy over clinical ecology, and is not easily answered, in fact many scientists would argue that no connection can be made unless some test can show an objective reaction, either by skin testing or changes in antibody levels in the blood or some other measurement such as hair analysis. Unfortunately the state of the art does not as yet permit a conclusive test, but even in the absence of one it seems as though orthodoxy is now becoming more impressed by the results of treatment which, like homoeopathy, are individual and thus not easily reproduceable on a large scale.

One possible explanation of the mode of action was first documented by physiologist Hans Selye in his work on stress adaptation. Selye described three stages which an animal goes through after physical, chemical or immunological stress. It first goes into a state of reaction in the form of some degree of shock, when adrenalin circulates, then within a variable time gradually adapts to the new circumstances, during which it is reliant on cortisone from the adrenal cortex, but finally exhausts itself and enters a phase of inability to adapt as the supplies of cortisone are exhausted. It is this final phase of exhaustion, often brought about by intervening disease, childbirth or trauma which often acts as the precipitating factor for symptoms which had previously been unexpressed. This would explain why foods which had been tolerated for years, even to the point of addiction, suddenly become noxious.

Such a scenario may even apply to babies who, at the moment of birth, are extremely vulnerable to infection and so are donated a large supply of IgG and IgA antibodies through the mother's milk. Because IgA particularly is contained in the secretions of the gut it may provoke a reaction to an antibody swallowed by the baby, and manifests as the all-too-familiar colic. This may happen after the baby is introduced to new foods, around the age of three months, or even occur whenever the breast-feeding mother has eaten a particular type of food.

If food intolerance is suspected then an elimination diet is recommended as the most direct means of establishing the connection, as it is seldom possible to tell from a dietary history alone. All food should be eliminated for a period of five days, and only mineral water permitted to drink. At the end of this time different foods should be reintroduced one at a time, preferably beginning with those which have been on the menu since homo sapiens came down from the trees, such as fruit and meat, and only introducing grains and dairy products later.

SUSCEPTIBILITY AND THE HLA SYSTEM

The T lymphocytes have an awesome responsibility in recognising whether or not a substance is foreign to the body, and subtle errors of judgement result in certain types of disease processes. To help them to keep track of which cells are of their own kind, most of the cells in the body are, as it were, 'stamped' with a particular configuration of proteins as an antigenic marker on the cell membrane. Thus each person has a unique set of markings (except for uni-ovular twins who share the same stamp) and as these were first discovered on the leucocytes they are known as the Human Leucocyte Antigens or *HLA system*. In order to produce this stamp one of the chromosomes in the cell nucleus sets aside four spaces (called A, B, C and D) on each of which a specific antigen is inscribed rather like the PIN number on a cashcard. This has two particularly significant consequences.

The first is in the field of susceptibility to disease. It has been noted that the sufferers of some conditions are likely to have a certain type of HLA antigen. Thus people with psoriasis are likely to possess antigen number 6 at position C, so they are said to possess HLA C6. Similarly rheumatoid arthritis is associated with HLA D4 and both diabetes (the juvenile onset variety) and coeliac disease with HLA D3. In some diseases the association is only slight, but in others it approaches 100%. For instance 96% of patients with ankylosing spondylitis have HLA B27, and 85% of coeliacs HLA D3. This does not mean that these antigens in any sense cause the disease, indeed there are many who have a relevant HLA antigen who never display symptoms, but it does give us a much better model for understanding the concept of susceptibility within a measurable framework. A useful by-product of the presence of these antigens is their assistance in coming to a diagnosis, especially in the early stages of a disease when the symptoms may be unclear, as the presence of absence of an HLA antigen will be a significant pointer in one direction.

Another use of the knowledge of the HLA system is for the matching of organs and tissues before transplantation. Organ transplantation has only become possible hand in hand with advancing knowledge about immunology, and it seems that the closer the match of the HLA antigens on the four positions, the less likely rejection is to take place. Tissue-typing is now routinely performed and hopefully at least two and perhaps three of the four antigens can be matched – the key does not have to fit perfectly in the lock to turn it! As was said before, some tissues have more HLA antigen than others, consequently corneas are relatively easy to graft, kidneys moderately so, heart and lungs more difficult and the liver hardest of all.

CANCER

The body reacts to malignant tumours in its tissues in the same way as it does towards grafts – by rejecting them. It is able to do so because a healthy immune system recognises cancer cells by the abnormal antigens which they carry, called 'tumour specific antigens', which mark them out for destruction. The process of 'cancering' appears to be happening all the time as mutating cells throw up primitive forms at periodic intervals, but this is of little consequence as long as they are swiftly discovered and destroyed. It is only when a defect in the immune system allows one of these potentially independent tissues to escape control that the 'disease' of cancer is said to have occurred. So it is obvious that cancer cannot be transmitted from one person to another by injecting them with malignant cells. Indeed, there are those who consider that the immune system in mammals developed as much for a safeguard against these internal dangers as to combat threats from the environment in the form of micro-organisms.

A dramatic example of this occurred in 1968 in America when one of the early kidney transplants was being performed. Unbeknown to the surgeons the donor kidney contained a very early cancer and when a routine postoperative chest X-ray was performed some weeks later the attendants were startled to see several rapidly enlarging secondaries. Surmising that these could only have come from the kidney, this was re-explored and indeed found to contain the primary tumour which had taken advantage of the immunosuppressive drugs used to prevent graft rejection. There was no alternative but to remove the donated kidney and stop the drugs, whereupon the lung secondaries rapidly regressed and the patient recovered.

Once a tumour has established itself, it may relentlessly go on to destroy the body but this is unusual. More commonly a balance is reached in favour of the tumour but the immunological mechanisms fight a rearguard action and slow its growth, sometimes even reversing it. The outcome largely depends upon the ability to revitalise the ailing immune system which allowed the tumour to occur in the first place. For this reason removing the primary site of growth may actually sometimes increase the rate of spread of secondary metastases because it was the primary tumour which was stimulating a reaction in the immune system. However, this is by no means always the case, and sometimes the secondaries regress or are slowed down.

The inability to eliminate colonies of malignant cells increases with age and hence we see a higher incidence of cancer in the elderly who tend to have an impairment of their cell-mediated immune system. We also see a higher incidence in those tissues and organs of the body which are exposed to a multiplicity of antigens during their lifetime and this may explain why the tissues of the lung, breast, stomach, colon, cervix and skin, which are in constant contact with potential allergens, are therefore more liable to cancer.

IMMUNE DEFECTS

Such a complexity of operations is involved in the protection of the body that it is perhaps hardly surprising that one breaks down from time to time and we are left vulnerable to any passing micro-marauder. On rare occasions children are born with a defect in the system and no immunoglobulins are made, so that once the maternal antibodies are lost they rapidly die of infection at the age of six months. More commonly defects are acquired in the course of time, and until the arrival of the condition we call AIDS this was usually the result of tumours of either the lymphocytes or the plasma cells, and known as Hodgkin's disease or multiple myeloma respectively.

Hodgkin's disease is a form of cancer involving the T lymphocytes which are located in the lymph nodes and the spleen, and is seen mostly in teenagers and young adults, especially men. There is painless swelling of the lymph glands in the axilla, neck and chest, and these small, rubbery swellings later enlarge to a considerable size and extend to the other lymph tissues in the body, including the marrow to cause anaemia. At the

17

beginning of the disease there is sometimes a fluctuating fever every few days, and the person may wake with night sweats and sometimes general itching of the skin. An unusual and very significant feature is pain in the bones or the glands coming on after drinking alcohol. There will usually be a significant loss of weight too. With treatment the prognosis is very good and over 80% survive. A similar condition called *lymphoma* or 'non-Hodgkin's lymphoma' occurs in older people and is rather more malignant.

Multiple myeloma is a cancer seen mostly in the elderly and involves the *plasma cells* derived from B lymphocytes in the bone marrow, which produce huge numbers of a particular 'runaway clone'. These proliferating plasma cells are all of the same type and therefore manufacture vast amounts of the same IgG antibody, far more than the body requires. A large mass of plasma cells develops in the marrow and causes nagging, deep pain in the bone and often a spontaneous fracture. The cells metastasize and take over other sites in the marrow, so the skeleton becomes studded with multiple areas of cells which crowd out the other developing cells leading to anaemia, thrombocytopenia (lack of thrombocytes) and neutropenia (lack of neutrophils).

The results are the clinical symptoms of bruising and infection so characteristic of the disease, and death from pneumonia or some other infection is common. The blood is so overloaded with IgG from the huge numbers of plasma cells that it spills over into the urine but cannot be seen unless the urine is heated. This makes a useful diagnostic test for the disease, as by warming a specimen of urine a cloud of 'Bence-Jones protein' appears, but then redissolves when the urine is brought to boiling point.

ACQUIRED IMMUNODEFICIENCY SYNDROME (AIDS)

Fear, sex and righteous indignation are the preferred ingredients of a good headline as any journalist will tell you, and the condition of AIDS has been billed for all three. It has come to occupy a corner of our mind previously reserved in the Victorian era for syphilis and in the middle ages for the Black Death, and represents the greatest public health challenge the human race has yet had to face. In the eight brief years since the pandemic began, huge amounts of time and human resources have been surrendered to the urgent need to prevent the spread of the disease, as it became increasingly clear that a rapid cure or immunisation was nowhere on the horizon.

Many of the initial speculations which arose have been answered with facts, and the speed with which information has dispersed has meant that patients are in some cases better informed than their doctors. But there is still a misunderstanding that the diagnosis is equivalent to a sentence of death, and many myths abound concerning the progress and outcome of the condition. All in all the outbreak has severely undermined the optimistic assumption that drugs and vaccines are the ultimate solution to all human ills, and one of the fringe benefits of the outbreak is a reclamation of responsibility for one's own health.

The Virus: AIDS first came to the attention of the medical world in San Francisco in 1981, where an unusual number of gay men were admitted to hospital suffering from a rare type of pneumonia caused by the parasite *pneumocystis carinii.* Subsequent investigations showed that this was brought about by a defect in their immune system which was grossly depleted of T lymphocytes, and thus allowed so-called *opportunistic infections* to take place. Much speculation abounded at the time about the origin and manner of spread of the disease, and the search for a virus was instigated when antibodies were found in the blood of patients suffering from the disease as well as in some of their contacts.

A virus was indeed isolated in the blood of a carrier in 1985, by both a French and American team, and later given the name human immunovirus 1 (HIV1). In retrospect it was found that an AIDS-like illness had taken place in an area in Central Africa three years previously, and serum taken from these patients at the time was now discovered to contain the virus. It seems that the virus had a ten year start in the African population, which is reflected in the very high incidence of the disease there today. Moreover, in West Africa the prevalent virus, termed HIV2, is of a slightly different strain, and closely resembles the simian variety of immunovirus (SIV) found in monkeys. Did humans catch the disease from apes, or have both groups derived it from a third source? No-one is sure.

The Epidemiology. For the first seven years the epidemic in the West has increased exponentially, but there is now evidence that the rate of spread is slowing down, especially among the gay population which bore the first impact of the disease. The number of people with AIDS in the UK at the time of writing is about 1,000, with an estimated 60,000 who are HIV positive (i.e. have been in contact with the virus). The numbers break down to approximately 70% gay or bisexual men, 25% intravenous substance abusers and the remainder either haemophiliacs who have been given unheated blood products or heterosexual contacts.

The mode of spread is virtually entirely by blood to blood contact, in a manner similar to that of hepatitis B. Only minute abrasions in the skin are sufficient for the virus to gain entry, and the rectal mucosa is very fragile and liable to abrade easily, so blood contact is highly likely to happen. It may, however, occur less easily during vaginal intercourse, as

19

well as by intravenous injection with unsterilised equipment (IV drug users), bleeding gums (transmission to dentists), needle stick injuries (nursing staff) and untreated blood products (haemophiliacs and those who sustain emergency operations in ill-equipped hospitals in Africa).

There is no evidence that the disease has been contracted via mosquito bites, although this might seem a distinct possibility. Nor is it known to have been passed through kissing, although the virus has been shown to be present in saliva, as well as in breast milk and seminal fluid. In these circumstances the amount is so small as to reduce the risk to virtually zero, moreover the virus is quickly inactivated by hot water or detergent.

Recently a second generation of the infection has come about because of babies who have contracted the disease in the womb. The virus is able to spread across the placenta and affect the developing embryo, and the tragic figure of neonatal AIDS is now being seen among young children in many parts of the world.

Seroconversion is the name given to the reaction of the body to the presence of the virus, in the course of which antibodies to the protein coat of the virus are made. This process does not happen at the time of contact with the virus, but takes about two to three months, during which time there is a possibility of passing on the disease without being aware of having it. In fact it is around the period of seroconversion when the individual is at his or her most infectious, and blood banks have to be extremely careful to assess their potential donors as the 'AIDS test' will not be positive yet.

At or shortly after the time of infection there may be a short flu-like illness in some, in others this takes the form of a more prolonged incapacity resembling glandular fever, with sore throat, swollen glands and painful joints. Almost always recovery from these episodes is complete, and a minority have neither of the above.

There then follows an interval when one is 'body-positive' but has no untoward symptoms that anything is amiss. It is impossible to attempt to speculate on the duration or the outcome, and the statistics are misleading, but so far approximately one third of HIV positive individuals develop symptoms of AIDS within ten years. The likelihood of this happening does depend very much on one's individual constitution and general health, as well as the promotion of a positive attitude toward life. However, for some the road can be a difficult one sometimes fraught with patterns of ill health, the main ones being termed PGL and ARC.

Progressive generalised lymphadenopathy (PGL) is a chronic, lingering continuation of the glandular fever-like illness mentioned earlier. The main characteristic is the enlargement of the lymph glands of the axillae and neck. There is a headache, aching muscles (myalgia) and a feeling of weakness, indicative of the ongoing struggle between the body's cellular defences and the virus. The virus cleverly tries to circumvent the defence by presenting an antigenic protein from its coat to the macrophages, which then surround the virus particle. There then follows a mutation on the part of the virus, which allows it to escape the retribution of the antibodies and remain safe within one of the main defendents of the body.

AIDS-related complex (ARC) is the name given to the onset of additional symptoms indicating that the virus is multiplying and gaining the ascendent. As well as the swollen glands, a recurrent fever develops with characteristic night sweats and loss of weight. Anaemia is likely to be present and recurrent attacks of diarrhoea. It is at this point that early opportunistic infections may manifest, such as sore throats caused by the presence of herpes of candida.

The full-blown picture of **AIDS** which may eventually emerge is most commonly heralded by *pneumocystis carinii pneumonia* (PNP) which manifests as a cough with a little sputum and severe shortness of breath. Sometimes some blood is coughed up, and there is a wheeze. Other opportunistic infections can also cause a cough, especially TB, herpes simplex pneumonia and cytomegalovirus (see chapter 3). About one third develop a rare form of skin tumour – *Kaposi's sarcoma* – which is seen as patches of dusky pink discolouration especially on the palate, and which gradually becomes more swollen.

Because the virus has been phagocytosed by the macrophages it is able to use these to gain admission into the nervous system by using these 'Trojan Horse cells' to infiltrate the normally impervious blood–brain barrier. There it causes a form of encephalitis in about 30% of patients, which can be very variable in its severity. It may only be a very subtle change in cognition with slight forgetfulness and slow thinking, but in others it causes a major breakdown in ability with confusion, difficulty conversing and eventually loss of consciousness.

Drug therapy and AIDS. Much effort has been extended to finding a drug which would be able to destroy the HI virus by some means, or at least slow down its rate of reproduction and T-cell destruction. The virus uses an enzyme called *reverse transcriptase* to make a DNA copy of its RNA for replication, and as there is no human equivalent of this it would appear to be an obvious target. Some sixty preparations have been tried without real success, but one, termed zidovudine (Retrovir/AZT) was shown in a trial to reduce or at least postpone the chances of developing PNP by a large degree. It has therefore been licensed for general use, but there is unfortunately a high price to pay in terms of unwanted effects. About half of the patients taking it develop anaemia, some severe enough to require a blood transfusion, and usually a low white cell and platelet count also, as well as headaches, nausea and weakness.

The other allopathic approach is to give prophylactic drugs to prevent the onset of opportunistic infections, mainly PNP, which is the main cause of death, and for this two drugs are chiefly used. The first is one which has been in use for very many years, Septrin (see chapter 3), whose side-effects are uncommon and well-known. The other is termed pentamidine and is given usually as an inhaled aerosol spray three or four times a day. It, too,

TABLE 2.1	Possible causes of lymph gland enlargement
Condition	**Pointers**
Local Enlargement:	
Tonsillitis	Fever, sore throat, occ. quinsy
Infected wound or abscess	Usually obvious
Cellulitis	Spreading red rash nearby
Rubella	Occipital glands, rash, conjunctivitis
Malignancy	Gland painless and hard
Lyme disease	Tick bite, arthritis
General Enlargement:	
Glandular fever	Fever, sore throat, sometimes a rash
Hodgkin's disease	Glands rubbery, not painful, itching
Toxoplasmosis	Large spleen, cat contact, fever
Cytomegalovirus	Fever, transplant history
Secondary syphilis	Rash, previous ulcers on genitals
PGL (AIDS)	Night sweats, weight loss, diarrhoea
Leukemia	Anaemia, bleeding, infections
Sarcoidosis	Wheezing and breathlessness

has side-effects, mainly a sore throat and bronchus, sometimes some wheezing and occasionally more serious effects like hyoglycaemia and even kidney damage.

AUTOIMMUNE DISEASE
It was an early axiom of immunology that the body could never injure

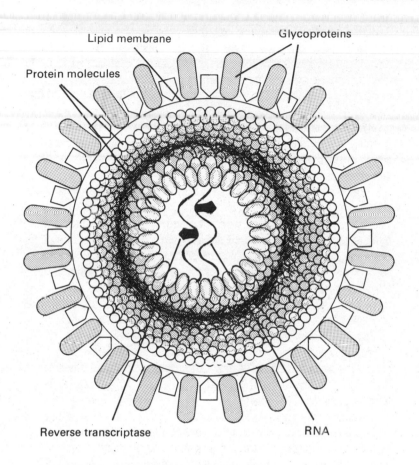

Lipid membrane

Glycoproteins

Protein molecules

Reverse transcriptase

RNA

FIGURE 2.2   *The AIDS virus*

itself in any way and that the immune system was unable to turn against itself. All the evidence, however, indicates that on certain occasions it will do just that. In fact we have already seen how the tissues of the lungs and gut may at times over-react and lead to self-inflicted injury in the form of allergies, although these are in the main restricted to the surface of the body. It appears that under three separate circumstances the body engages in a form of civil war which expresses itself as one of the 'autoimmune diseases'.

The first of these, and the most common, is the group of organ specific autoimmune diseases in which cells from a secretory gland are disrupted for some reason and leak their contents into the blood. There they come into contact with the lymphocytes which read them as foreign, since they have previously been screened from any contact, and go on to make antibodies against them, which can be detected by examining the blood. This antibody reaches the gland and sets about destroying it, so that eventually it atrophies and a deficiency disease results. The glands involved are the thyroid (Hashimoto's disease), the stomach lining (pernicious anaemia), the pancreatic beta-cells (insulin dependent diabetes), the hair follicles (alopecia), the salivary glands (Sjogren's syndrome) and many others.

The second situation is rare, affecting about one person in 20,000, and results in a condition called *systemic lupus erythematosis* (SLE), so-called because of the prominent red, saddle-shaped rash on the nose reminiscent of the stripe of a wolf (lupus = wolf). SLE had been known for years as a condition of young women leading to kidney failure, arthritis and other systemic malfunctions, but the cause remained a mystery until strange deposits of immune complexes were noticed in the kidneys and these were found eventually to be antibodies against the nuclear material of the body's own cells. It seems that normally the nuclei of cells are well hidden from the immune system, but on occasions break down to release large molecules of DNA which act as antibodies, and the ensuing immune complexes block any small vessels in the body and cause inflammation there, so the disease runs a prolonged course until kidney failure usually terminates matters.

A rather different type of autoimmunity occurs where the antigen of an invading organism happens to be identical to that of one of the host's own tissues, with the result that the antibody formed, having seen off the invader, then goes on to set about its own organs. Once again, it is the glomerulus of the kidney which is often selected, as well as the synovial membrane of the joints and the tissues of the heart. The results take the form of the diseases which are known as *acute nephritis* and *rheumatic fever* and are discussed in the relevant chapters.

CHAPTER THREE

INFECTION:
DISORDERS OF
SUSCEPTIBILITY

THE CONCEPT OF INFECTION

The Industrial Revolution which transformed Europe brought with it a series of epidemic diseases which swept into the overcrowded cities and ravaged the populations. These took the form of cholera, typhoid, smallpox, diphtheria, scarlet fever and TB, and medical opinion was divided into three opposing theories about the cause and spread of infectious disease – the contagionist, the miasmatic and the zymotic. The contagionists held that minute particles were spread through food and water, and that these multiplied in the body as 'animalcules'. The miasmatists felt that disease was the result of noxious gases which they called 'miasms' (although not quite the same as what Hahnemann, the founder of homoeopathy, meant when he referred to miasms), and that these arose from decaying matter. The zymotic theory considered that each infectious disease was the result of a specific ferment or 'zyme' and that they were passed by contact from one body to another. All these ideas had something of the truth, but were unable to shed any light upon prevention of infection. It was only by isolating the sufferers for a period of forty days in quarantine (Fr.quarant=forty) that some control over the spread of smallpox could be obtained.

Into this arena came two men who were to change opinions, the German pathologist Virchow and the French bacteriologist Pasteur, and both were able to make use of the microscope which had been invented two centuries before by the Dutchman van Leeuvenhoek, but which had only recently been sufficiently developed to view what came to be known as 'microbes'. Virchow believed that all disease was fundamentally a result of cellular abnormality, and to that extent he is often considered the father of pathology. His view was that under normal circumstances the cells in a healthy body are able to adapt to changes which might in others lead to disease, and he emphasised susceptibility, believing that microbes were largely the by-product of disease rather than its cause, although he never denied their existence. Pasteur, however, was able to demonstrate the microbes and also to prevent the outbreak of certain diseases by the use of his vaccines, and the medical and pharmaceutical professions have since tended to his view rather than emphasising susceptibility and prevention. In fact most of the decrease in the infectious diseases were due to social, environmental and dietary improvements and took place before the advent of antibiotics and mass immunisation.

THE MICRO-ORGANISMS

Only a few of the vast numbers of the different types of micro-organisms are actually involved in humans in any way, and of these the majority are commensals, that is they lead a symbiotic relationship but do us no harm and may even be beneficial. This is particularly true of bacteria, and many parts of the body possess their own colonies which tend to preserve the status quo and resist the spread of *pathogenic* or harmful bacteria. Viruses are, of course, very much smaller and live within the cells where they multiply, so if they do so much damage that the host dies, they are left without a home. For this reason viral infections tend to be less dramatic and more prolonged than bacterial. Much larger than both of these, but still invisible to the naked eye, are the smallest animals, the *protozoa* (such as amoebas) and the plants lacking chlorophyll, the *fungi,* which are also involved in certain disease processes. Much larger species than these are the insects and worms which infest, rather than infect us, and which are easily seen with the naked eye and therefore not technically micro-organisms at all.

To compare the enormous range of size involved, let us assume the average human cell to be the size of a refrigerator. A red corpuscle will be as big as a car tyre, and a bacterium a football. Viruses will vary in size from a grape to a pea, depending on the type. In the other direction a protozoon will be the size of a packet of cornflakes or larger, while the multicellular organisms like lice and worms will be the size of a large field and a small town respectively.

VIRUSES

Because of their minute size (they are the smallest living creatures), viruses could not be visualised directly until the invention of the electron microscope in 1937, but long before this their existence had been assumed because of the ability of an unknown 'poison' (the Latin word for poison is 'virus') to pass through filters which remove bacteria. Finally some of the substance was crystallised and found to be composed partly of either RNA or DNA, the nucleic acids of which the genes in the nucleus of the cell are made. It was then realised that a virus reproduced by taking over the duplicating apparatus of the nucleus and substituting its own blueprint, so manufacturing its own kind and finally killing the cell. Because the essential ingredients of the virus were virtually identical to those of the host cells, this meant that any form of chemical destruction by the newly-invented antibiotics was out of the question and it was only the body's ability to form antibodies that prevented capitulation.

Viruses are involved in many of our commonest infectious diseases. The common cold has variable symptoms and may be a result of the activities of any of four different families of viruses, of which one, the rhinoviruses, has over a hundred members. Those viruses containing DNA are in the minority, and form the herpes family, the wart or papilloma viruses and the smallpox virus.

The RNA viruses are associated with such conditions as influenza, measles, mumps, rubella, diarrhoea, pneumonia, meningitis, hepatitis, polio and rabies. One group in particular, *respiratory syncytial virus* or RSV, invades the respiratory tract of babies, who develop bronchitis and pneumonia at an early age, usually in the winter months of their first year and who may become severely ill. Another seasonal condition of babies is 'epidemic winter vomiting', in which there is vomiting and diarrhoea, often with dehydration, and in whom the wheel-shaped *rotavirus* appears in the stools. The *arboviruses* are so-called because they are transmitted by insects that live in the jungles (L.arbor = tree), particularly mosquitoes (yellow fever, dengue fever) and ticks (viral encephalitis). The *enteroviruses*, which live in the gut but exhibit symptoms elsewhere, include that of polio (the virus damages the nerve cells of the anterior horn of the lower spinal cord, thus paralysing the legs) and of the *Coxsackie virus* associated with hand foot and mouth diseas (Coxsackie is a town in New York State where the virus was first isolated.)

THE HERPES FAMILY

Of all the hundreds of viruses trying to make a living on the human race, none are more successful or enterprising than the herpes viruses (Gr. herpo = to creep). They have acquired the ability to hibernate for long periods inside a cell, sometimes for the whole of the host's lifetime, and break out when conditions are right to spread to others. Four groups of human herpesviruses are known:– herpes simplex (cold sore), herpes varicella/zoster (chickenpox and shingles), Epstein-Barr virus (glandular fever) and the cytomegalovirus (CMV).

Herpes simplex is responsible for symptoms in a variety of different areas of the body but the basic lesion is always a blister. The initial attack, when the virus first establishes itself in the body, occurs either in the region of the face or the genitalia as a rule, and two slightly different strains of the virus are involved, herpes simplex I or HS1 *(herpes labialis)* in the mouth and HS2 or *herpes genitalis* on the genitals. The method of transmission is by contact, either oral for HS1 or sexual for HS2, and during the primary attack the symptoms are often so mild as to pass unnoticed. In some, however, the first attack is severe and there may be *stomatitis* with mouth ulcers, especially in young children. Occasionally the virus selects an unusual site, such as the cornea to cause a *dendritic ulcer* (see chapter 19), or the finger to cause a herpetic whitlow, or even a very unpleasant generalised infection of skin which is previously eczematous – *eczema herpeticum*.

Once the primary infection is over, the virus travels to a site on a nearby nerve ganglion where it remains in a dormant state until reactivated by a stimulus such as trauma, sunlight, cold or intercurrent illness. HS1 has a preference for the trigeminal ganglion, and when reactiviated travels down the trigeminal nerve to a site on the face, usually the lips as they are more vulnerable. Here the virus irritates the cells to cause the familiar tingling sensation, followed by a blister which then crusts over and slowly heals. During the stage of blister-formation the virus can be passed to another person by direct contact, and in fact 19 people out of 20 actually carry the virus, although many are unaware of it.

HS2 is slightly different, in that it has a preference for the sacral nerve ganglion and produces identical ulcers on the penis, labia or cervix, which are painful and often multiple. In the event of cervical lesions, there will usually be a discharge and some generalised malaise and fever, and recurrent attacks damage the cells and predispose towards cervical cancer. Moreover, if a woman with active cervical herpes gives birth, there is a chance that the baby may develop a generalised herpes infection which is often fatal, and sometimes a Caesarian delivery will be recommended.

Herpes varicella/zoster (VZ) is the cause of both chickenpox and **shingles**. Chickenpox, described in more detail in the next section, is the primary infection of the virus and it is only when this reactivates that it produces the condition known as shingles, or herpes zoster. Once the child has recovered from chickenpox, the virus remains dormant in a cranial or spinal sensory root ganglion and may years later may produce a blistering, red, painful rash over the area of distribution of the nerve, typically the ophthalmic division of the trigeminal nerve to involve the eye or forehead. Or a small area of the trunk or abdomen supplied by a single nerve root may be affected forming a band around the body, 'a belt of roses from hell!'. If the attack is a severe one the blisters may later become deep scars and remain continually painful, *post-herpetic neuralgia*, and this is especially likely to occur in the elderly. Because the blisters of shingles contain the active virus, it is possible to contract the primary form of the disease – chickenpox – from a case, but not vice versa.

Glandular fever is a condition found mostly in teenagers and young adults though sometimes it may be the cause of an unexplained fever in younger children. Labelled the 'kissing disease' by the popular press, it is indeed mostly passed on by salivary contact, and has an incubation period of anything from 1 to 4 weeks and does not cause epidemics but rather isolated cases. The cardinal symptoms are a fever, sore throat and swollen glands, so that initially it is very similar to acute tonsillitis with which it is easily confused. However, the course of glandular fever tends to be a protracted one, going on for months in many cases, with chronic weakness, headaches and lack of interest in life.

Some other features by which the disease can be distinguished are the appearance of swollen glands in other parts of the body, small red spots on the hard palate, stiffness and swelling of the joints in some cases, and sometimes a transient rash on the body and puffiness around the eyes. In about half the cases there is enlargement of the liver or spleen, leading to mild hepatitis and even sometimes severe enough to cause jaundice.

In order to confirm the diagnosis blood can be sent for examination of the lymphocytes, and these are seen to have abnormally large, misshapen nuclei and be present in very large numbers (hence the American name for the disease *infectious mononucleosis*). These cells are formed as a response to the presence of the *Epstein-Barr virus*, the source of the trouble. The EBVirus also stimulates the production of antibodies, and these can be detected by a test called the monospot test.

Cytomegalovirus or CMV is an example of what is sometimes called an 'opportunistic infection', that is it does not cause symptoms unless there is a considerable lowering of the resistance of the host, when it is able to seize the opportunity. It is therefore most often seen in those patients who have had transplants and are immunosuppressed, or in those suffering from cancer or AIDS. They develop a condition similar to that of glandular fever, with hepatitis and even pneumonia. The name 'cytomegalovirus' derives from the enlarged cells seen in tissues infected with the organism.

CHILDHOOD ILLNESS

During the months following birth a baby is protected from the majority of infectious diseases by the presence of maternal antibodies. By the age of about 6 months, however, these will have been lost by the natural process of degeneration and the infant will therefore be to some degree susceptible to infection. Once the infection has been contracted, the person will thereafter usually have lifelong immunity from that particular disease, although rarely they may get it twice.

Most childhood diseases are of viral origin, and spread through the community by droplet infection from coughing, or sometimes by actual contact (contagion). Only rarely are they contracted by water-borne or food-borne methods, except in the case of gastroenteritis which is discussed separately. Following the acquisition of the organism there is a period of a few days while it multiplies within the body to form sufficient numbers to cause symptoms, the *incubation period*. Towards the end of the incubation period, which differs in length according to the disease, there is a rise in temperature and general loss of well-being, before the onset of the symptoms specific to the disease itself, and this is known as the *prodromal period*.

Because the child is infectious during the prodromal period, and sometimes during the incubation period as well, the condition is quickly passed around the community, and small epidemics occur which if widespread and affecting other countries are known as 'pandemic'. Whether or not an epidemic occurs depends largely on the level of immunity of the majority of the child population, and when this falls below about 50% then a new one is likely to break out, which happens every 4–5 years or so. In between some isolated cases occur but there are an insufficient number of susceptible individuals around for the organism to establish itself.

Measles is associated with a virus and responsible for an enormous morbidity and mortality worldwide, especially where the host is in a poor state of health initially. It is responsible for 1% of total world deaths and is especially devastating in Africa. The virus affects chiefly the skin and respiratory tract, and is transmitted by droplet infection, having an incubation period of about 12 days. Children aged between 1 and 5 years are mostly involved, the first symptoms being non-specific fever and catarrh with a dry, croupy cough – the *catarrhal phase*. These are indistinguishable from a cold unless the mouth is examined, when the presence of *Koplik's spots* can be seen like small grains of sand on a deep red background opposite the molars on the mucus membrane of the cheek.

A day or two later the rash appears, the *exanthematous stage*, usually on the forehead and behind the ears as a pink, slightly raised series of small blotches. This spreads to the face and trunk, and less commonly the limbs. As it does so the spots become larger and confluent (joined together), lasting 4–7 days and then fading with slight scaling. There is accompanying *conjunctivitis* with watering and redness of the eyes which is mild but causes some photophobia (hence the old wives tale about light damaging the eyes). The main complication of measles is *otitis media* and the slight risk of perforation of the drum which seems to lead to chronic discharge in some. The *bronchitis* which is part of the disease may sometimes turn into a more severe chest infection with pneumonia, especially in the undernourished or immunosuppressed. Rarely, in about 1 in 1000 cases, there is progression to encephalitis after a week or so, and the patient becomes stuporose and convulsions may occur.

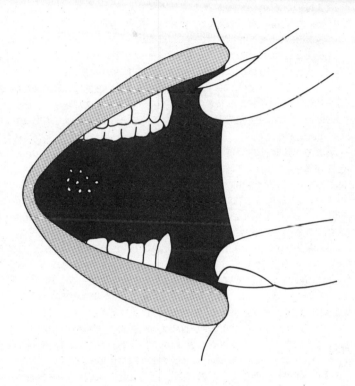

FIGURE 3.1   *Koplik's spots*

Rubella or *German measles* is an altogether milder condition and although the symptoms are similar in some ways to measles it is an unrelated virus. In about half the cases the rash does not appear or goes unnoticed as it is so brief, which is why many people have antibodies to the virus but are unaware of ever having had the disease. The remainder develop a mild prodromal phase with malaise and fever for a day or two, after incubating the virus for about 2–3 weeks, and then a faint, pink rash appears mostly on the trunk, but not as marked as the dusky blotches of measles. The rash lasts from a few hours to a few days, and there is often redness and watering of the eyes, and enlargement of lymph nodes of the neck, especially those in the occipital area, and sometimes in other parts of the body too. In older girls and women there may be some stiffness of the joints which can persist for months, especially in the fingers or the knees, but eventually resolves without complication.

The main danger of rubella is when it occurs in mothers-to-be in the first three months of pregnancy, when the cells of the foetus are differentiating to become the different organs and are very susceptible to the virus at this stage, particularly the heart and nervous system. This may result in congenital abnormalities such as heart lesions, deafness, cataract or mental handicap, especially if the infection was acquired within the first month of pregnancy (when the mother could even be unaware that she is pregnant). For this reason there is a policy to offer rubella immunisation to girls at an early age.

Mumps is a glandular infection, again of viral aetiology, spread by droplet infection in the same way as measles and rubella. Here the incubation period is longer, about three weeks on average, followed usually by swelling of the salivary glands, most commonly one of the parotids but sometimes it may start in the submandibular. The gland is tender and swollen, and salivation may be uncomfortable so the pain is worse at mealtimes. If the inside of the muth is inspected the red orifice of the parotid duct may be seen in a position very close to where Koplik's spots (see under measles) would be observed, beside the molars. Swelling of the salivary gland lasts a few days and then subsides, perhaps going to another or to the testes, ovaries or pancreas.

Quite a number of children experience some abdominal pain due to a mild degree of *pancreatitis*, and about 20% of post-pubertal boys experience inflammation of the testis (*orchitis*), although only a very few, about 1%, develop sterility afterwards. A benign form of *meningitis* is sometimes seen as the glandular symptoms are resolving, when the child will complain of severe headache, drowsiness, neck stiffness and perhaps stupor. There may also be photophobia and vomiting, so any of these symptoms should alert one to the possibility. Fortunately the condition resolves without damage and most children make an uneventful recovery within about a week.

Chickenpox or herpes varicella is a generalised febrile illness which may be caught by droplet infection or by contact with a blister of either another case of chickenpox or a case of shingles (which is the same virus appearing at a later stage). The incubation period is about two weeks, following which flat spots or *maculae* appear on the trunk and sometimes the face and mouth but seldom much on the limbs. These soon progress to lumps or *papules* and then swell with clear fluid to form tiny blisters or *vesicles*. As these are very itchy they are generally scratched and become infected, so the clear fluid becomes pus (*pustules*) and finally scabs over and disappears, often leaving a scar crater, the whole process taking about a week. As well as the skin lesions the patient suffers from a general illness with headache, fever and limb pains, but these symptoms disappear as the crops of spots clear up, generally after about a week.

When chickenpox occurs in an adult it is usually of a more severe nature and the illness is more prolonged, with the risk of complications such as *varicella pneumonia* which develops within a few days of the eruption of spots, leading to a cough and sometimes haemotysis. A form of *meningitis*, similar to that complicating mumps, may appear, but in this case is likely to be more severe and possibly leave permanent damage, particularly to the cerebellum causing ataxia (staggering). The complication of *shingles* has already been mentioned in the previous section.

Recently an indirect complication of chickenpox in particular has been described in children who are given aspirin for the fever. Known as *Reye's syndrome*, it is very uncommon but has a high mortality in the few who are afflicted by it, and may leave those who recover with a degree of brain damage. The drug causes damage to the liver and brain and produces symptoms of vomiting, drowsiness and eventually deep coma. Reye's syndrome is also seen in children with influenza and less often in other febrile illnesses, so it is now recommended that aspirin is never given to children with fevers.

Roseola is a very mild and only slightly infectious illness of infants and young children, and a virus is suspected but has not been identified. The incubation period is about 12 days and is followed by a slight fever and as this vanishes a faint, pink, macular rash appears on the neck and trunk lasting only a few hours. There are no complications to this common illness, and it is so similar in appearance to a mild case of rubella that the diagnosis is often unconfirmed.

Fifth disease is called such because it is the fifth of the viral childhood fevers to exhibit a rash. Another name, which describes it more aptly, is *slapped cheek disease*, because of the very characteristic bright red rash on the cheeks, which spreads gradually and more faintly to other parts of the body over a few days. The child is not unduly ill, but, like rubella (with which it is sometimes confused) it tends to lead to some stiffness of the joints, especially the fingers.

Whooping cough is unlike most of the other childhood diseases in that it is probably caused by a bacterium, bordetella pertussis, rather than a virus and the symptoms continue for a considerable time, often amounting to several months. The condition is caught by droplet infection from someone in the catarrhal stage and this is followed by an incubation period of about 7 days. The first evidence of illness is a runny nose and loose cough with slight fever, indistinguishable from a cold, but after a week or so this *catarrhal phase* changes to the *paroxysmal phase* as the mucus thickens and the infection descends into the lungs to plug the small bronchi.

Great effort is required to expel the sticky mucus, and this causes the typical paroxysms of coughing followed by the inspiratory 'whoop' so typical of the disease. The spasm of coughing leads to cyanosis, salivation and often vomiting, occasionally with convulsions if there is sufficient lack of oxygen. Because of the very high pressure generated in the thorax by coughing, the eyes bulge and may even haemorrhage. Hernias occasionally develop and even rectal prolapse. In between the attacks the child is able to breathe normally without coughing, and it is only in babies and young children that the disease is usually serious. Gradually the severity of the symptoms lessens, but a cough will often persist for months afterwards.

The complications of pertussis are uncommon but occasionally some sticky mucus will plug a bronchus completely so that the lung beyond it will collapse, a condition called an *atalectasis*. A *lung abscess* can then form in the stagnant tissue, or a secondary *pneumonia* may occur. If the bronchi or their cilia become locally damaged, they tend to dilate and form small pockets of residual infection and a continuing disability termed *bronchiectasis* (qv) is the result. However, serious neurological reactions, such as may follow pertussis immunisation, are very rare.

Scarlet fever is another illness where bacteria play a part, in this case a particular strain of *streptococcus* (see next section). This was once a greatly feared disease, running swiftly through communities and families and often rapidly fatal. Today it is a pale shadow of itself, possibly because the bacterium has undergone mutation, and the term *scarlatina* is sometimes used instead. After an incubation period of 2–3 days the child develops a high temperature and a sore throat, often with enlarged tonsillar glands and infected tonsils. The next day a red rash like a flush starts behind the ears and spreads to involve the whole body, sparing the area around the mouth ('circumoral pallor') as the muscle here is attached firmly to the skin. The redness is caused by a toxin secreted by the streptococcus. The tongue is initially furred, the 'white strawberry', but then peels to leave the typically 'red strawberry' tongue at the same time as the rash on the body fades and peels over a period of a week or so.

The two possible complications of scarlet fever are *rheumatic fever* and *acute nephritis*, both of which are rare but are described in the sections on heart and kidney disorders respectively.

TABLE 3.1	Showing the number of days for which a person should be regarded as infectious
	Periods of infectivity
Measles:	FROM the onset of the catarrh UNTIL 4 days after the onset of the rash
Rubella:	FROM 7 days before the rash UNTIL 4 days after the start of the rash
Mumps:	FROM 7 days after the first swollen gland appears
Chickenpox:	FROM three days before the onset of symptoms UNTIL the rash has started to scab
Pertussis:	FROM the first catarrhal symptoms UNTIL about three weeks after the start of the illness
Scarlet fever:	VARIABLE, depending on duration of throat symptoms, the infection can be passed even though the patient is symptomless
Glandular fever:	FROM a week before the onset of symptoms UNTIL a week after the onset

BACTERIA AND THE BODY

Bacteria, although larger than viruses, cannot really be classified in either the plant or animal kingdoms. They contain only a single chromosome in a primitive nucleus, and have a rigid cell wall which determines their shape. This shape is an important factor in classifying bacteria, and takes the form of spheres (*cocci*), rods (*bacilli*) or spirals (*spirochaetes*). In a bacteriology lab much time is spent incubating bacteria on plates of nutrient agar jelly, upon which colonies will readily grow given suitable conditions, and this gives information of their presence in food and water supplies as well as in the body. Unlike viruses, many bacteria are able to survive for long periods in adverse conditions by hibernating as spores, rather like the seeds of a plant.

The cocci, when examined microscopically, like to group themselves into either clusters if they are *staphylococci* (Gr.staphys = bunch of grapes), in rows if they are *streptococci* (Gr.streptos = chain) or in pairs if they are *diplococci*, such as the gonococcus and the meningococcus.

Staphylococci are the great pus-forming organisms, pus being the debris of phagocytes and dead bacteria, and they are therefore seen in *boils, abscesses, styes, wound infections, impetigo* and many other conditions, including *food poisoning*. The reason for the latter is that some varieties of staphylococci also secrete a toxin which has a severe effect on the gut. There are many different members of the family, some quite innocent which live on the skin, and some potentially pathogenic (harmful), often living in the nose. It is from here that they may be shed to cause skin infections and boils in the susceptible (which is why masks are worn in hospitals), and many are resistant to some antibiotics such as penicillin from whose clutches they escape by producing an enzyme, ß-lactamase, which destroys it. Occasionally staphylococci gain entry from a skin infection into the blood, and a septicaemia or blood-poisoning occurs with the possibility of metastatic abscesses forming in other parts of the body, such as the joints, lungs or bones.

A condition known as the *toxic shock syndrome* is thought to arise from the invasion of a particular strain of staphylococcus through the vaginal wall if it has been damaged or dehydrated, usually through the use of modern super-absorbent tampons. This leads to sudden collapse during the menstrual period with a high fever, diffuse red rash with severe diarrhoea and vomiting. The patient is often confused and shocked and may be severely ill for several days.

Streptococci produce large numbers of different toxins – enzymes which destroy the body's defences in some manner. One of these works by breaking down the cement which holds the cells together, enabling the bacterium to spread rapidly under the skin (as in cellulitis and erysipelas). Another operates by producing an 'erythrogenic toxin' which causes the red rash seen in scarlet fever and the 'strep throat'. Many varieties of streptococci are able to break up or 'haemolyse' the red blood cells, and this is used as the basis of their classification into different groups named the Lancefield groups.

Streptococci are involved in such various conditions as *tonsillitis and sore throats, scarlet fever, otitis media, lobar pneumonia* (in the form of the pneumococcus) and *puerperal fever*. They appear to have moderated their behaviour towards humans in the last few decades, however, in that they are by no means as virulent probably because of mutation. They are also usually very susceptible to penicillin and less likely to produce resistant strains.

Following an infection with one particular streptococcus, the Lancefield group A variety, an individual may subsequently develop one of three separate conditions due to the production of antibodies which unfortunately act against the body's own tissues. These tissues are the heart, particularly the heart valves, to cause rheumatic fever, the glomerulus of the kidney to cause *nephritis*, and the skin of the legs to cause the characteristic blotchy rash of *erythema nodosum*.

The *diplococci* are bean-shaped bacteria which tend to exist in pairs. The two chief disease-causing diplococci are the *gonococcus* which is associated with gonorrhoea and can be seen in the urethral or vaginal discharge of cases of this disease, and the *meningococcus*, seen in the cerebrospinal fluid of cases of bacterial meningitis. Recently both have developed a considerable degree of resistance to many antibiotics.

The Bacilli. There are numerous very different rod-shaped members of this genus, a few of which, like the tetanus and gangrene organisms, are able to survive anaerobically without the need for oxygen and live in the soil and decaying matter. These are members of the family *clostridium*, some of which, notably the botulism bacillus, produce the most powerful poisons known.

Most bacilli, however, require oxygen to survive, such as the mycobacterium family which are known as *acid-fast bacilli* because of their ability to resist strong acids, and which comprise the leprosy and tuberculosis organisms. A much larger family is that of the enterobacteria or *coliforms* because they live in the gut. They include bacillary dysentery, typhoid, plague and of course the well-known E.coli which causes problems especially if it strays into the urinary tract. Other bacilli are the comma-shaped vibrio of cholera, the whooping cough bacillus and brucellosis.

Spirochaetes. These spiral bacteria are best known for their relationship with *syphilis* and *yaws* (a tropical disease very similar to syphilis), and these types are known as Treponema. Another type of spirochaete, Leptospira, is seen in a severe form of jaundice found in canal and sewage workers – *Weil's disease* or *leptospirosis*.

Chlamydia. As well as the three main groups of bacteria, there are several groups of rather smaller organisms which fall midway in size between bacteria and viruses. One of the better known of these is the chlamydia, a furry little beast named after the Latin 'chlamys' meaning a hair shirt, and thought to be involved in the condition known as *non-specific urethritis* or NSU, the commonest form of sexually transmitted disease. The very same organism also features in certain eye conditions under the name of *inclusion conjunctivitis* seen in children after they have been swimming, or in adults who may acquire it indirectly from the genital tract. The eye disease *trachoma* is probably its most notorious manifestation world-wide, and is a common cause of blindness in Third World countries (see chapter 19).

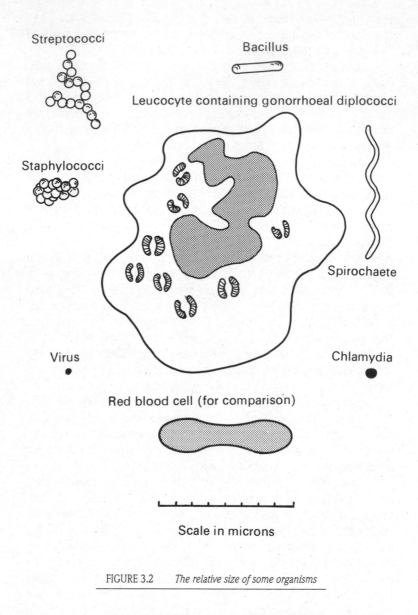

Streptococci

Bacillus

Leucocyte containing gonorrhoeal diplococci

Staphylococci

Spirochaete

Virus

Chlamydia

Red blood cell (for comparison)

Scale in microns

FIGURE 3.2   *The relative size of some organisms*

Another form of chlamydia occurs in the form of *psittacosis*, one of the so-called 'atypical pneumonias' and seen in those who handle certain birds, particularly parrots, budgerigars and ducks.

DIARRHOEA AND GASTROENTERITIS

The digestive tract, like the respiratory tract, is constantly in contact with the environment and is thus liable to contamination by allergy, poisoning and infection. The reaction of the body is to attempt to rid itself of the offending substance, which it does by vomiting and diarrhoea, common symptoms of all types of 'food poisoning'. Infections are seen particularly in countries where hygiene and water-supplies are inadequate, often resulting from parasites such as amoebas and giardias whereas antibiotics are the main cause of such symptoms in the West. Nor is it usually possible to distinguish chemical from infective causes from the nature of the symptoms alone, and consideration of the diet is necessary. However, as treatment is largely a question of replacement of the fluid lost, the distinction is mostly irrelevant.

Diarrhoea in Babies and Infants

In young babies gastroenteritis may lead rapidly to dehydration if severe, and this causes a succession of symptoms. Initially they are restless, pale and thirsty and pass only a small volume of urine. As the fluid loss progresses the skin shrivels and loses its elasticity and the tongue becomes dry. Eventually dehydration and loss of electrolytes from the blood and tissues causes the infant to look very gaunt, with sunken eyes and fontanelles. By this time the child is severely ill, and may become cyanosed and collapse, so intravenous fluid must be introduced before this stage is reached.

Severe attacks of gastroenteritis occasionally occur in neonatal wards, caused by a pathogenic strain of E.coli that secretes a dangerous toxin. Normally a harmless gut commensal, it is spread rapidly during nursing procedures and carries a high mortality. Babies and infants are also liable to rotavirus infection which occurs in sporadic outbreaks as *epidemic winter vomiting*, a flu-like illness often accompanied by a cough and a cold as the virus also inflames the respiratory tract.

Even after the acute illness has been overcome the cells of the small intestine are left damaged and unable to produce the enzyme lactase needed to digest milk, so when this is reintroduced into the feed the stools remain loose and frothy. Milk should therefore be avoided for 2–3 weeks after severe diarrhoea until the *lactase deficiency* has been restored.

Sometimes other infections such as *otitis media, pneumonia or meningitis* may present as diarrhoea or vomiting, and evidence of these conditions should be looked for.

Diarrhoea in Children and Adults

In this age group diarrhoea is often mild and due to an inappropriate diet

Bodyweight Lost %	Symptoms
TABLE 3.2	Showing the Symptoms of Dehydration
2	Thirsty, irritable, restless
5%	Scanty urine, pale, rapid breathing
7%	Dry mouth, sunken eyes & fontanelles, lax skin
10%	Stuporose, limp

or sometimes an enterovirus ('gastric flu'). Certain foods such as undercooked red beans, poisonous fungi, shellfish and mackerel contain potential poisons which may give rise to symptoms. Food which has begun to decompose will form amines called ptomaines, and before the advent of refrigerators this was a common source of food poisoning.

Staphylococcal food poisoning may follow the consumption of food contaminated with these organisms, which are present on the skin of an infected food-handler and which contain a tasteless toxin which is resistant to heat, so that the toxin may still exist even though the bacteria have been killed. It is this type of food poisoning which leads to the sudden severe stomach cramps experienced by aircraft passengers, for instance, when a whole batch of food becomes contaminated by the organism. The symptoms, though dramatic, seldom last more than 24–48 hours, and there is no accompanying fever. A similar toxin-mediated condition is caused by *bacillus cereus*, a bacterium which has a preference for re-heated cooked rice and is sometimes an unwelcome extra in a take-away meal.

Consuming infected meat or milk may result in a condition named *campylobacter enteritis* after the organism involved. Outbreaks occur particularly in schools or are contracted from pets, and are characterised by a slow onset of fever, nausea, muscular pains and abdominal pain, sometimes confused with appendicitis. This is followed by profuse, offensive and often bloodstained diarrhoea the next day which may be so severe as to cause incontinence and may last for several weeks.

Salmonella gastroenteritis is another condition seen after consumption of infected food, especially meat and poultry, and is becoming increasingly common. The usual way of contracting it is through frozen produce which has not been thoroughly heated while cooking, or from the handling of food by a salmonella carrier. Symptoms are sudden diarrhoea, usually with vomiting, fever and colicky abdominal pain, and sometimes severe illness with shock and dehydration in the elderly. About 5% of sufferers continue to harbour the organism in the gallbladder after they have recovered, and excrete it in the stools as carriers.

Diarrhoea in Travellers

Those who travel to certain parts of the world are at increased risk of infection from organisms in the locality, as well as from the alteration of their diet which may in itself cause symptoms. So-called *traveller's diarrhoea* (Delhi belly, Montezuma's revenge) is a result of contact with a strain of E.coli with which the gut is unfamiliar but which is local to the area and therefore does not cause symptoms to the indigenous population. The diarrhoea is sudden, usually mild and self-limiting after a few days once the intestine has become colonised. Although often labelled 'dysentery', this name should really be reserved for a different disease related to the bacillus Shigella (*bacillary dystentery*). The shigella species come in different types, some of which are quite virulent and cause the life-threatening bloody diarrhoea of the tropics such as Kipling describes so vividly, while others are involved in a relatively mild disorder.

Cholera was once a relatively common European disease despite being known as the 'Asiatic cholera', but is now only seen in certain areas of the world, mostly the Ganges basin. The comma-shaped vibrio periodically mutates and spreads in world-wide pandemics, of which we are now in the seventh, El Tor, variety. Spread is through the contamination of drinking water by sewage as a rule, and when this is drunk then a few days later there may be abdominal pain and severe watery diarrhoea in enormous volume ('rice water stools'), so most deaths come from the inevitable dehydration. The reason for this is that the vibrio secretes a toxin which prevents the intestinal cells from absorbing any salt or water, thereby losing it from the body.

Typhoid and *paratyphoid*, collectively known as the **enteric fevers**, are not primarily diarrhoeal disorders but it is convenient to discuss them here. Both are due to varieties of salmonella, but the illness is generally much more severe and prolonged. Like salmonella, it can be contracted from carriers directly but more often is a result of consuming infected food or water. The bacteria can survive gastric acid and then penetrate the wall of the intestine to get into the lymphatics from where they are spread all over the body in the blood stream. This results in the typical symptoms of fever with rigors, headache and a dry cough, often with abdominal pains also, and then as the illness progresses the rose-coloured spots appear on the skin and the spleen becomes enlarged. It is after this that the diarrhoea starts, by which time the patient is extremely ill with weakness and mental confusion, and there is a risk of the bowel perforating and causing peritonitis.

Two forms of diarrhoea found commonly in tropical countries are caused by protozoa which exist freely in both food and water, and to which the local population are to some extent immune. *Amoebic dysentery* starts as a diarrhoea with colicky pains and abdominal distension, and may become chronic despite treatment, when the diarrhoea continues or may become persistant constipation. The amoebas colonise the lower bowel from where they are liable to travel in the portal system to the liver and there form multiple abscesses ('amoebic hepatitis'), but this is not a common complication. They may also cause permanent damage to the gut wall which becomes stripped of its villi with the result that malabsorption occurs, a condition which is still sometimes known as 'tropical sprue'.

Giardiasis is another protozoal condition, caused by Giardia lamblia, which also occurs in temperate countries such as Britain and the USA. Unlike amoebiasis, this is a parasite of the small intestine and the symptoms are therefore mainly nausea, flatulence and distension after food, as well as less severe diarrhoea. The organism is water-borne and lives in the bowel of sheep and deer who have contracted it from humans. In undernourished children it may become chronic and destroy the villi of the small intestine to cause malabsorption (see chapter 13), but does not travel outside the gut.

ANIMALS, INSECTS AND INFECTIONS

In order to propagate itself successfully an organism needs not only a host but also a successful means of transmission. This means, in effect, a choice between droplet infection from one pair of lungs to another, intimate physical contact (most commonly of a sexual nature), food or water carriage or, most ingeniously of all, by means of a third party to act as a go-between. This will usually require a fairly complicated adaptation to life in more than one species, and is seen especially in some of the present day tropical diseases as well as in the great plagues of history. Mosquitoes (malaria, yellow fever), ticks (typhus, Lyme disease), snails (bilharzia/schistosomiasis), rats (plague, Weil's disease), cats (toxoplasmosis) and even parrots (psittacosis) are examples of the variety of possible vectors. Most of these are uncommon in the developed world, but every so often an outbreak will occur and re-emphasise our proximity to nature and the animal kingdom.

It was in 1975 that there occurred an outbreak of arthritis among the children of the small town of Lyme, Connecticut who were noticed to be generally unwell with severe headaches and flu-like symptoms for several weeks. This was given the name **Lyme disease** and started a search for possible linked causes, and it was not long before suspicion fell upon the fact that most if not all of the victims had been bitten by an insect found later to be a tick which is commonly found in the long grass of the area and is spread by deer. The bite causes a slowly enlarging area of redness on the skin as the spirochaetes which have been inoculated begin to multiply, and eventually they reach the local glands which swell and become painful. More seriously, unless adequately treated, the disease causes neurological damage with meningitis and paralysis of the cranial nerves, and often leads to swollen, painful joints. The disease has now spread to most parts of the USA, as well as to Europe and the UK, and there is a small (about 5%) risk of contracting the infection after tick bites.

Another condition which is prevalent world wide and on the increase is **toxoplasmosis**, which has recently gained notoriety for its glandular fever-like symptoms, although the organism is totally unrelated to the EB virus of glandular fever. It is in fact a protozoon and spreads to humans from cats, in the intestines of which it reproduces itself. The cat excretes the cysts and these are spread either direct to humans through cat litter trays and gardens, or else ingested by other animals such as goats, sheep and pigs. Thus drinking unpasteurised goat's milk or eating undercooked mutton or pork can lead to the disease with its chronic sore throat, headaches, swollen glands and fever.

The particular risk of toxoplasmosis, however, is to pregnant women and their foetus if sustained in the first three months of pregnancy, when it is often subliminal. They will commonly sustain a miscarriage, but if not the foetus has a 40% chance of developing congenital toxoplasmosis. The brain and retina of the baby is most often affected which may at first be symptomless but progress after some months to cause visual damage or worse.

Also on the increase in the UK is the illness which on a world scale is responsible for the highest mortality – **malaria**. This now causes some 1500 cases a year in this country, almost all contracted abroad, and should be suspected in a traveller who develops a high and intermittent fever. Several types of the malaria protozoon exist in the world, all transmitted by mosquito bite, but the most dangerous and resistant is the falciparum variety endemic in sub-Saharan Africa.

The protozoa are taken up by the liver where they multiply for about two weeks (hence the need to continue treatment after return home), and are then released into the blood. At this point the fever begins, only to subside when they invade the erythrocytes for the purpose of replication, which takes two to four days depending on the type of parasite. Thus malaria is described as *tertian* or *quaternary* depending on the interval of the fever which only occurs when the organisms are released, and is seen as a rapid rise in temperature accompanied by rigors (uncontrolled shivering).

Each time the parasites re-invade the blood cells the fever subsides, only to return with a vengeance after the specified period. Because many of the red cells are contained in the spleen, this organ becomes inflamed and swells to a great size (*splenomegaly*). In some species the progression is very rapid, and the rupture of the erythrocytes as the parasites emerge causes widespread *haemolysis* (see chapter 8). The haemoglobin spills over into the urine where it is seen as the dreaded 'blackwater fever', and also clogs the capillaries of the brain to cause cerebral malaria with coma, and those of the kidneys to cause renal failure.

TABLE 3.3	The possible causes of fever
Associated features	**Possible causes**
Cough	Flu, bronchitis, pneumonias, sinusitis, TB, whooping cough
Rash	Childhood fevers, meningitis, glandular fever, typhoid
Diarrhoea	Gastroenteritis, meningitis, Legionaire's dis., hepatitis
Aching muscles	Flu, ME, Polymyalgia rheumatica, malaria, glandular fever
Painful urination	Pyelonephritis, Bright's disease
Weight loss	TB, Hodgkin's disease, PGL, malignancy, endocarditis, thyrotoxicosis
Altered consciousness	Meningitis, Legionaire's dis
Painful joints	Rheumatic fever, rheumatoid arthritis, Lyme dis, rubella, glandular fever, septic arthritis, SLE
Recent travel	Malaria, typhoid, Weil's disease

Perhaps the best clinical description of malaria has been by Hippocrates, who wrote in the *Epidemics*:

"Philiscus, who lived by the Wall, took to his bed on the first day of acute fever; he sweated and towards night was uneasy. On the second day all the symptoms were excacerbated; late in the evening had a proper stool from a small enema; the night quiet. On the third day, early in the morning and until noon, he appeared to be free from fever, but towards evening acute fever with sweating, thirst, tongue like parchment, passed black urine, night uncomfortable, no sleep, he was able, no sleep, he was delirious on all subjects. On the fourth day all the symptoms were worse, the night more comfortable, urine of a better colour. On the fifth day about midday, had a slight trickling of blood from the nose, urine varied in character, having floating in it round bodies resembling semen. A suppository having been applied some scanty flatulent matters were passed, night uncomfortable, talking incoherently, extremeties cold and could not be warmed. Urine black, loss of speech, cold sweats, extremeties livid. About the middle of the sixth day he died. The respiration throughout like that of a person recollecting himself, was rare and large, the spleen swelled up, the paroxysms on the even days."

INFESTATIONS

As well as the micro-organisms there are two groups of animals which may infest the skin and intestines of man – the insects and worms respectively. Although often irritating and sometimes debilitating, they seldom cause serious disease but may be difficult to eradicate as the immune system is unable to make antibodies against them.

The **scabies** mite is spread by close, often sexual, contact between people, and burrows under the skin to cause intense itching, particularly at night when the warmth encourages the mites to move about. The lesions tend to start in between the fingers and on the wrists, sometimes in the groin area. Later they travel to other parts of the body and no part is exempt. On close inspection the tiny burrows made by the mite can be seen, terminating in a blister, although if scratching is severe these become obliterated and a widespread rash may result which can be misleading so that any generalised itchy rash should make one suspicious. If the scratching is severe it may frequently result in secondary skin infections or impetigo (qv). As well as using an insecticide to destroy the mites (which should be repeated after three days), the clothes and bedding must also be well washed to prevent reinfection.

Lice are another form of insect parasite but live only on the hairy parts of the body, different varieties being closely adapted to certain areas and races, even to the extent of having specially shaped claws to cling to the hair of different races. Pubic lice or *crabs* are found in the pubic hair and, like scabies, are spread mostly by sexual contact. They may also travel to other parts of the body such as the axillae or even eyebrows but not the hair on the head which is the province of head lice, usually seen in schoolchildren. The eggs of the head louse are found around the nape of the neck as small grey *nits* attached to the hair about halfway along, and these take about two weeks to hatch so the treatment must be repeated after a fortnight as only the lice are killed.

Threadworms are also mainly seen in children who ingest the eggs in contaminated soil, often through chewing their fingernails. The eggs hatch in the intestine after two weeks or so, and the worm emerges from the anus at night to lay eggs on the skin, causing irritation of the area as it does so. The scratching causes contamination of the fingers and if these are not washed the whole cycle starts again. On occasions the threadlike worms, about half an inch long, are noticed in the stools, sometimes even in those of family pets who may harbour the parasites.

Tapeworms are much less common in this country since meat has been under closer scrutiny at the time of slaughter, as most cases arise from infested pigs or cattle who contain the worm in their gut. The tapeworm head attaches itself to the wall of the intestine and grows in a series of segments to many feet in length. Periodically a few segments detach themselves and are excreted as short pieces of white ribbon which can be seen in the stools. Most symptoms arise from the colicky pains and loss of appetite that the tapeworm causes.

ANTIBIOTICS

No drug has revolutionised the practice of medicine and the expectations of patients more than penicillin and the subsequent torrent of derivatives and analogues which followed it. Prior to 1940 the outcome of infection depended largely on the vitaltiy of the individual and the skill with which this was supported. To day it is assumed that for any infection there is somewhere an antibiotic solution, and death, if not exactly optional, is at least culpable.

The serendipity discovery of penicillin is well known. Fleming was culturing some bacteria in his laboratory at Cambridge, while simulta- neously Florey was investigating the mould penicillium on the floor above. Neglecting to cover a dish of bacteria overnight, he was surprised to find many of them dead the next day where some of the spores of the mould had landed, and an industry was born. Since that day soil bacteria and moulds have been a fruitful source of antibiotics and antibiotic precursors, and the great majority have come from bacteria themselves. Many of these have been chemically adapted from their natural forerunners in order to get rid of unwanted effects or add further attributes.

Before penicillin the only allopathic drugs used extensively against bacterial infection were the sulpha drugs, which inhibited bacterial growth by blocking the synthesis of folic acid which bacteria need in great quantities in order to reproduce. Of these only one, Septrin, remains widely used today, and this is used mainly in urinary infections and more recently to prevent pneumocystis pneumonia in HIV positive individuals.

At one time the elements mercury and arsenic were used but both of these produce extremely toxic side-effects.

Pencillin had the advantage of being bacteriocidal, that is it actually killed the bacteria rather than preventing their reproduction and awaiting their removal by the body's own defences. It was also extremely effective against most of the cocci, but did suffer from several drawbacks. Firstly it was very rapidly secreted through the kidneys which meant that it had to be given often, and then by injection as the acid in the stomach destroyed it. In fact, during the post-war period, supplies were so short that the drug had to be recovered from patients' urine and re-used! The most serious problem, however, was its tendency to cause an anaphylactic reaction (see chapter 2), with devastating results.

To overcome these defects, the penicillin nucleus was chemically synthesised and then modified to give derivatives which have improved over the years. The current one, *amoxycillin* (Amoxil), has a somewhat broader spectrum than penicillin (i.e. it is active against a greater range of bacteria), is not destroyed by acid and so can be given by mouth, and lasts much longer in the body. The pharmacists, however, have not had it all their own way.

The greatest ally which bacteria possess is time. While it takes humans 20 years to reproduce a generation, bacteria can replicate in 20 minutes and thus compress the equivalent degree of evolution of half a million generations in one human lifetime. This has enabled them to develop resistance by virtue of their chance mutations, a feature which the use of antibiotics encourages by killing off their competitors, the non-resistant ones. This applies especially to penicillin, against which they have bred an enzyme, *beta-lactamase*, which inactivates the drug, so the latest range (Augmentin) is now augmented by a beta-lactamase inhibitor.

Although the penicillins are still the most widely used antibiotics, many other groups have beeen explored. One of the first of these was *tetracycline*, found in 1948 in a sample of soil, and active against a wide variety of organisms – the first of the *broad spectrum* antibiotics. For many years it was the mainstay against respiratory infections, where a large variety of organisms are found, but increasing resistance has decreased its success even with some of the modern derivatives. It is still in common use, though, mainly against the smaller bacteria, chlamydia and some viruses against which it has partial success, as well as against some less common infections such as brucellosis, leptospira, psittacosis and Lyme disease.

Another antibiotic group, the *cephalosporins*, were first discovered in Mediterranean sewage and a great many varieties have been developed.

47

They also have a broad spectrum and are less likely to cause hypersensitivity than penicillin, but are much more expensive.

Finally, mention must be made of two commonly used antibiotics which are given for certain protozoal and fungal infections. The first of these, *metronidazole* (Flagyl), is almost the only drug capable of suppressing protozoa such as amoebas and giardias, as well as killing the bacteria seen in pelvic and vaginal infections. It has several possible unwanted effects, such as nausea, headache and dizziness, but is particularly unpleasant if taken with alcohol. The other is the antifungal drug *nystatin* (Nystan) which is active against candida in the gut and vagina, as well as other yeast infections on the skin.

Altogether almost 100 antibiotics are listed in the British National Formulary, the majority of which are duplicates or used only in highly specialised situations ranging from TB to osteomyelitis. Like the armament industry, we hope that we never need to use them but are nevertheless glad they exist just in case. The wholesale destruction of populations of any kind can have long and short term repercussions, however, which are both unpredictable and hard to assess. Nature, it is said, abhors a vacuum, and by destroying our commensal organisms we can never be certain what will take their place.

CHAPTER FOUR

SKIN:
DISORDERS OF
PROTECTION

Our skin is much more than just an impervious envelope enclosing the body, it is a complete organ in itself, in fact the largest sense organ in the body. Its other functions include controlling body temperature, screening the suns rays with the pigment melanin, insulating the body with a layer of fat, manufacturing vitamin D, secreting certain unwanted substances and signalling our emotional states by flushing (whether we like it or not). There are even areas of specialised skin – the hair and nails – for different protective functions, and one or more of these may malfunction in a variety of ways.

Skin disorders are numerous and many reflect more general abnormalities of the body, signifying the presence of internal disease. They are perhaps best analysed according to the tissues affected and the underlying contribution which the make. Most of the symptoms of skin disease fall into the categories of a discoloration or rash, an itch (which is actually a mild form of pain), or a swelling of some kind.

THE ECZEMAS

The term eczema literally means 'to boil over', and well describes the irritation and redness that takes place in the various forms of this condition, of which there are several types.

Atopic eczema is perhaps the best known, being a largely inherited predisposition to such allergic states as asthma and hay fever. It is thought that there is a transient deficiency in the local immunoglobulins in the gut mucosa during the first few months of life, which is when atopic eczema often starts, and that this allows food allergens to enter the blood and cause widespread stimulation of other antibodies which are situated in the epidermis. This partly explains the low incidence in breast-fed babies. Atopic eczema is usually worst in the skin creases of the elbows, knees and wrists (which is why it is sometimes known as *flexural eczema*), but it is also seen on the face, neck and trunk. By the age of 10, about 90% of children will have cleared up apart from the most severe cases. If the eczema is scratched it may become infected and develop *secondary impetigo*, and if an eczematous child contracts a cold sore he or she is liable to have a widespread and dangerous eruption wherever there is eczema (*eczema herpeticum*).

If a particular area of skin is scratched incessantly it will become thickened and rough, and is then described as having become *lichenified*, a term used for a number of disorders where the epidermis comes to resemble lichen. *Lichen simplex* or neurodermatitis is such a type of thickened eczema localised to one area of skin which is abraded incessantly either through habit (e.g. the neck or wrist), or because of sweating (pruritus ani & vulvae) or even localised atopic eczema. It is seen especially in overstressed individuals as a well-defined ridge of purple skin.

A similar situation occurs in *varicose eczema* where the underlying irritant is blood leaking from dilated varicose veins around the ankles, which discolours the skin a dull slate-grey and dries it up, leading eventually to cracking and ulceration.

Pompholyx eczema (Gr.pomphos = bubble) occurs mainly in young adults, especially those whose hands and feet sweat. It generally starts on the sides of the fingers as small, itchy, symmetrical blisters and may spread to the palms or soles before drying out and cracking to form chronic fissures. In most cases it is due to exposure to chemicals and detergents during housework etc, but in some is a reaction to fungal infections of the feet or to the ingestion of excess nickel found in some stainless steel pans.

Not all inflammations of the skin are eczemas, occasionally large blisters appear on the epidermis and in the mouth for no determinable reason and rupture to leave painful raw areas – *pemphigus*. Another inflammatory condition, more itchy than painful, is *lichen planus*. As the name suggests the lesions are raised and irregular, being a shiny pink or purple colour and found mostly on the wrists, shins and sacrum. They last for several months and then resolve, and are accompanied by a painless rash in the mouth consisting of a white, lacework pattern of spots and streaks which are of great help in diagnosing the rash.

DERMATITIS & URTICARIA

The skin responds to stimulation from chemicals, trauma, temperature change and some foods in a variety of ways, the chief of which are by becoming inflamed (dermatitis) or swelling up (urticaria). The terms 'eczema' and 'dermatitis' are often used interchangeably, but technically the word 'dermatitis' means the type of eczema which follows directly or indirectly from contact with a chemical substance, while 'eczema' should be reserved for the constitutional types described in the last section.

Dermatitis is the inevitable consquence of contamination of the skin by certain substances, such as bleach, cement, washing powders, certain oils and dyes, and a rash will appear within a short time if protection is not used. Nappy rash caused by the ammonia in urine is an example. Other substances lead to allergies which do not manifest immediately but appear as dermatitis a week or so later.

What happens in these cases is that following contact with the substance a small amount penetrates the skin and is passed to the local lymph nodes where antibodies are formed a few days later. The antibody then makes its way back to the epidermis and reacts with any remaining allergen it finds there to cause an area of irritation. In some cases the rash is more generalised and affects mostly the thinner skin of the eyelids, backs of the hands and fronts of the elbows to give puffiness and erythema (redness). When this happens the allergen may have long gone and be untraceable, but is commonly topical antibiotics or other creams, lanolin, rubber, chrome, nickel or plants such as primulas and poison ivy.

A special case, *photodermatitis*, is where the sensitised skin only reacts to the drug or other chemical where it is exposed to the sun, so the rash is restricted usually to the backs of the hands and the face. It seems that these substances enable sunburn to occur with even a small dose of UV light.

Urticaria is an itchy, blotchy, transient rash characterised by swelling of the skin or mucus membrane involved. This is brought about by an increase in the permeability of the vessels after histamine has been liberated in their vicinity, either by damage to the mast cells by allergens (similar to asthma) or by direct injection. Some types of food such as shellfish, strawberries, nuts, fish and a host of food additives may lead a few minutes or hours later to a general reaction in the skin which comes out in weals very similar to those caused by nettles but larger. Because the dermis rather than the epidermis is involved, the swelling is pronounced compared to dermatitis, and may reach very large proportions if the tissues of the lip, tongue, face, throat or eyelids are involved when the condition is sometimes referred to as *angio-oedema*.

Some, who are very susceptible, may go on to chronic urticaria when they are seldom free of the rash which comes on in response to physical stimuli such as cold, sunburn or pressure. There is likely to be sensitivity to certain foods and an exclusion diet may be needed to discover what can be tolerated. Not uncommonly they exhibit the symptom of *dermographism*, when stroking the skin will evoke a typical weal and flare response.

One specific type of urticaria, *papular urticaria*, also known as *heat bumps*, is that caused by the bites of insects, particularly fleas. The rash takes the form of recurrent eruptions of itchy papules all over the trunk which fade within a few days only to reappear infuriatingly after the next bite. The body has become allergic to the saliva of the flea, and usually it is the family pet that gets the blame although fleas commonly lurk in old furniture and carpets.

DISORDERS OF KERATINISATION – PSORIASIS

Normally the epidermal cells are continually being formed in the deepest layers and migrating outwards to be shed at the surface. As they develop they are becoming hardened by a protein called keratin which also causes the cells to die, and in places subject to continual wear such as the palms and soles and wherever *calluses* form, the keratin layer builds up a greater thickness for protection. If such a callus develops at a point of pressure on the toe it may press on the nerve below to cause pain and is known as a *corn*.

Psoriasis is a mysterious condition of unknown cause whereby the rate of keratinisation of the epidermal cells is greatly speeded up, so that instead of taking a month to reach the surface they accomplish it in a few days and in doing so the process of keratinisation is inadequate, and so the cells all stick together. The result is that the thickened skin has a silvery, scaly appearance and flakes off prematurely to leave a pink, patchy, map-like rash underneath. This may be very disfiguring but, despite the name (psora means 'to itch'), not usually especially itchy. The condition affects about 2% of the population to some extent, but rarely starts before the teens and usually improves with age. Sometimes emotional or physical trauma or infectious disease is the precipitating factor, and there may be a family history.

Favoured sites are the prominences of the elbows and knees, the sacrum and the scalp especially at the hair line around the edge, but nowhere is immune. It is often symmetrical on the left and right sides of the body, and may arise at the site of trauma or an operation scar, (the *Koebner phenomenon*). Because of the different manner of keratinisation of the palms and soles, psoriasis is uncommon here but in those in whom it does occur it resembles large sterile pustules, *pustular psoriasis*. One common complication in about half of the cases is damage to the nails, usually as small craters in the surface called *pitting*, sometimes as separation of the nail bed or distortion. About one in fifteen sufferers develop an arthritis in one or more joints, often involving the fingers – *psoriatic arthritis*.

Ichthyosis is an uncommon condition seen mainly in cold, dry climates in young children, in most of whom it is inherited. The skin takes on a dry, scaly, fish-like appearance (Gr.ichtheus = fish) which in some cases is associated with the condition of atopic eczema and causes itching of especially the face and upper arms where it is prominent. Attention should be given to the diet which may be deficient in nicotinamide. A similar condition called *tylosis* affects only the palms and soles which are greatly thickened ('hyperkeratosis').

SEBACEOUS DISORDERS – ACNE

The sebaceous glands secrete a greasy substance, sebum, on to the hairs of both body and scalp for protection not only against water but also to discourage fungal infections such as ringworm (which is why it is children who generally get scalp ringworm as their glands are less developed). The rate of secretion of sebum depends largely on stimulation from the sex hormones, especially androgens. Oestrogens tend to lessen the flow, which is why women often notice a fluctuation during their menstrual cycle, but the small amount of testosterone which they produce is sufficient to stimulate the glands.

Acne is one of the main consequences of seborrhoea (literally the flow of sebum), and occurs because the glands do not operate by secretion, but rather by allowing the cells of the lining to coagulate into a mass and form the sebum. The narrow opening through the hair follicle becomes blocked by debris, and this gradually changes colour until it is the familiar *blackhead* or *comedo*. The latter name derives from the assumption by the ancients that these were some kind of maggot which was eating into the flesh, and means 'a glutton'. If the problem is limited to these comedones then a few minutes in front of a mirror will do the trick, but unfortunately the accumulated sebum is an ideal medium for certain strains of bacilli which exist on the skin, and these multiply within the sebaceous gland to cause the familiar pustules or 'whiteheads' on the face, back and chest. In the most severe forms of acne the inflammation extends through the walls of the glands into the subcutaneous tissues to form pus-filled cysts which may coalesce, leading to severe scarring called *cystic acne*. Even young babies are not immune and their developing sebaceous glands may incur quite marked spottiness termed *infantile acne* which does, however, remit spontaneously after a few months.

Rosacea is a somewhat similar condition and at one time went by the name of acne *rosacea*, although it is doubtful now that the problem lies in the sebaceous gland, indeed no-one seems to be quite sure where it does lie. Nevertheless, the appearances are broadly similar with red pustules forming on the cheeks and around the mouth especially, sometimes moving to the forehead or nose. The skin takes on a flushed, mottled look with dilated, broken vessels and the peculiar fleshy swelling of the nose known as *rhinophyma*, seen only in men and usually ascribed

53

quite erroneously to intemperance. A complication of this condition, seen mostly in women, is chronic conjunctivitis and persistant redness of the eyes.

Seborrhoeic eczema is a term used to describe a type of red, scaly and somewhat greasy rash common in babies and the elderly and largely restricted to the scalp (where it forms a severe type of *dandruff*) or the body folds (where it is termed *intertrigo*). Again there is no evidence that sebum secretion plays a part in the aetiology of the condition, but the distribution on the scalp and the body folds might lead one to suspect this. It particularly affects babies in whom it is seen around the eyes as *blepharitis*, behind the ears, in the groins as a severe form of *nappy rash*, and on the scalp as *cradle cap*. Quite often it becomes infected with yeasts such as Candida, and the tell-tale sign is when small 'satellite lesions' appear at the periphery of the rash.

VIRAL INFECTIONS – WARTS

The epidermis reacts to many viruses by producing excrescences of tissue in the form of warts. Most of these viruses fall into the category of human papilloma viruses (HPV), the name papilloma being used for any kind of benign tumour of the skin, different sites being associated with different viruses. Nor does HPV only involve the skin, for it is found also on the mucus membranes of the genitals as genital or venereal warts.

The common warts seen on the fingers is a curious subject,

TABLE 4.1	Possible causes of a Rash	
With fever:		
General rash:	Measles, Rubella, Chickenpox, Scarlet fever, Glandular fever, Meningitis, Toxic shock syn.	
Local rash:	Shingles, Impetigo, Lyme dis., Rheumatic fever, Erysipelas, Cellulitis, Typhoid, Meningitis	
Without fever:		
General rash:	Eczema, Dermatitis, Psoriasis, Lichen planus, Drug rash, Thrombocytopaenic purpura	
Local rash	– face:	Acne, Rosacea, Herpes simplex, Impetigo, Slapped cheek disease
	– trunk:	Pityriasis rosea, Pityriasis versicolour, Lichen planus, Roseola
	– legs:	Erythema nodosum, Henoch-Schoenlein purpura
	– varies:	Scabes, Urticaria, Ringworm, Drug rash, Shingles

apparently plagueing some individuals for months while leaving others untouched, sometimes emerging at the site of an injury (the Koebner phenomenon again), and sometimes taking the very smooth appearance of a planar wart on the face. When situated on the sole of the foot it is termed a *verruca* or plantar wart and sometimes covers large areas with hard, thickened skin (*mosaic wart*), and is often painful as the pressure drives it deep into the dermis.

A different strain of virus is seen in the penile and vulval warts known as *condylomata acuminata* (literally 'pointed knuckles') because of their irregular cauliflower-like shapes. These are almost always spread by sexual contact and often appear at the same time as other venereal conditions; they are also a factor in the aetiology of cervical cancer.

Children in particular are liable to crops of pearly-grey, firm swellings on the face or trunk. These are *molluscum contagiosum*, a type of wart in which a much larger virus, the poxvirus, may be found and which contains thick, cheesy material which can be expressed through the tiny dimple which surmounts the top. These warts are usually 2–10 in number and are about the size of a split pea.

Pityriasis rosea is the rather exotic name given to a disorder which is thought to be due to a virus, and which often occurs in children. The word comes from the Greek meaning 'bran-like' and describes the speckled appearance of the fully-fledged rash. The first indication that something is happening is the apperance on the trunk of a pink, oval patch known as the *herald patch*, as it precedes the rash proper by several days. The child is usually perfectly well in himself and is often thought to have ringworm until the typical macular speckles appear on the trunk like an inverted Christmas tree, following the lines of the ribs. These last several weeks but eventually disappear leaving no ill-effects, nor is the child apparently infectious as the cases are invariably isolated ones.

BACTERIAL INFECTIONS – IMPETIGO

Large numbers of bacteria and yeasts populate the skin but seldom cause trouble unless there is underlying damage caused by sweating, scratching etc., when unwanted streptococci and staphylococci may arrive.

Impetigo is one of the more common consequences of either of these organisms and leads to a spreading infection of the epidermis when serum oozes from the raw and blistered surface and congeals as the typical honey-coloured crusts, moving about from one part of the body to another in a highly contagious fashion but seen especially around the mouth of children. It commonly follows the scratching caused by another skin condition such as psoriasis, eczema or scabes, and can be spread by fomites such as sheets, towels etc.

Some types of streptococci contain toxins which enable them to break down the connective tissue and spread rapidly across the skin as may happen in the *cellulitis* which follows some insect bites, and is extremely painful. When this happens to the tissues of the face this is termed *erysipelas* and leads to much oedema and swelling as the skin here is very loose and thin.

Staphylococci on the skin may inflame particularly the tiny glands attached to the hairs which secrete grease, and these then swell with pus. If this happens generally on the beard area it is called *barber's rash* or *sycosis barbae* as it is spread by shaving. Other parts of the body where hairs are found are liable to infection as *boils* or *styes*, and if the hair is removed they will discharge pus. If the boil is so large that it has several discharging orifices then it is called a *carbuncle*, and these kind of infections are particularly likely to occur in diabetics. Recurrent crops of boils (*furunculosis*) may result from malnutrition or poor diet, since the bacteria are able to reside symptomlessly in the nose and be spread by sneezing.

FUNGAL INFECTIONS – RINGWORM

Fungi are the most frequent unwelcome guests on our skin, usually those from the ringworm (Tinea) family. There are four main species involved with humans, and they seem to have their own preferred areas of activity.

Tinea pedis or *athletes foot* is pretty much restricted to the spaces between the toes in those who sweat profusely or are careless about drying themselves after a shower. The fungus is readily found on the floors of changing rooms etc. and in a few people will provoke a more general type of allergic reaction – the 'id' reaction – and cause irritation of other parts of the skin, including pompholyx.

Tinea corporis is seen on the trunk or limbs as a pink, raised area which gradually expands over a few days, clearing in the centre as it does so. This gives it the appearance of a ring similar to that formed by the 'fairy ring' of toadstools, and it is from this that the name *ringworm* derives (it was once thought to be an actual worm). In time satellite lesions appear around the edge, which helps to distinguish it from eczema, and the rash becomes itchy and is readily spread among schoolchildren. A very similar type of ringworm, *Tinea capitis*, can be caught from animals like dogs and cats and affects mainly the scalp. An inflamed and itchy area develops and the hair may be lost in a manner similar to alopecia from which it must be differentiated.

Lastly comes *Tinea cruris* or *dhobi itch*, which affects the area around the groin and armpits, and is caught in a manner similar to that of athletes foot, especially in the tropics. The name derives from the custom of Indian dhobis to wash the clothes in the nearest pond, and then starch them well which provided an excellent medium for the fungi and some embarrassing moments for the Raj!

TABLE 4.2	Possible causes of itching
Condition	Pointers
Skin disease	Eczema, psoriasis, scabies & many others
Old age	Common if skin gets dry
Jaundice (obstructive)	Gallstones, pancreatic tumour, drugs
Pregnancy (last trimester)	Abdominal mainly, may be iron deficient
Renal failure	Especially if uraemic
Hodgkins disease	Early stages especially
Coeliac disease	Rare, associated with dermatitis herpetiformis
Polycythaemia	After a hot bath
Diabetes mellitus	Rare, during onset of condition
Leukaemia	May be an early symptom
Drugs	Oral contraceptives, Largactil, many others

A fungus distantly related to Tinea may affect the skin of those who holiday in the sun and come back with an unusual tan. It is discussed in the next section under pigmentation disorders.

DISORDERS OF PIGMENTATION – VITILIGO
The colour of the skin is determined by the presence of the pigment melanin formed in the melanocytes of the basal layer of the epidermis. This dark brown pigment is extruded into the epidermal cells where it protects the sensitive nuclei of the epidermal cells from damage and possible malignant change from the ultraviolet radiation emitted by the sun. It is packed together more densely in those races who come from hot climates and who thus have a darker skin. The enzymes which produce melanin are activated by UV light, so exposure does tan the skin but as the epidermis is shed over the following weeks this tan goes with it. Nor is the current trend of exposing oneself more fully and more frequently to the elements without a certain risk of malignant change in later life, especially in the case of fair-skinned people in whom the melanin is distributed somewhat unevenly as collections of melanocytes better known as *freckles*.

Vitiligo is the patchy loss of pigmentation which is most obvious in coloured people to whom it may be a source of great embarrassment, not least because it superficially resembles the depigmentation seen in leprosy. The word comes from the Latin 'vitellus' meaning a calf and was used by the Roman physician Celsus to describe the resemblance ot the white spots on a calf's legs. The melanocytes in certain areas atrophy and even die leaving a widespread, symmetrical pattern all over the body. The condition is quite common, affecting about 1 person in 50 to some degree, and appears to be increasing. It is more common in those with autoimmune disorders such as pernicious anaemia and thyroid disease, and antibodies against melanocytes have been demonstrated.

A similar loss of pigment occurs for a completely different reason in *pityriasis versicolour*, and the two conditions are sometimes confused. However this variety of pityriasis is a fungal problem, arising on the neck and trunk of those who holiday in the sun, and leads to unexpected mottling of their tan until it fades. The acid produced by the fungus bleaches the melanin in small, localised areas and it tends to recur each year in the susceptible.

HAIR AND NAIL DISORDERS – ALOPECIA

Hairs consist of tubes of keratin which sprout from very active hair papillae at the roots where the cells are dividing at an enormous rate. This rate of growth is by no means always constant, however, and after growing to a length of 2–3 feet, which may take several years, the hair is shed and replaced by a new one. All this happens in a random pattern so that every day up to 100 hairs are lost from the head. In animals there is a more cyclical shedding which takes the form of moulting, but in humans this only happens after a severe illness, emotional trauma or pregnancy when there is a sudden thinning of the hair a few weeks later, followed by renewal.

Alopecia is the name given to patchy hair loss with well-defined edges (Gr.alopix = a mangy fox), and is seen on the scalp or beard area. It freqently starts in childhood but may occur at any age and the patches may be single or multiple and are usually about the size of a 50p piece. After a few months the hair generally starts to grow again but is often a lighter shade for a whlle. A few people develop alopecia of the whole scalp or even the whole body, in which case recovery is unlikely. Around the edge of the bald area are short, stumpy hairs with a swollen base – *exclamation mark hairs!* – which enable this condition to be distinguished from other causes such as ringworm of the scalp, hair pulling etc.

The cause of alopecia is thought to be an auto-immune process affecting the hair follicles and in some cases there is an association with vitiligo. It is also more common in those who have Down's syndrome.

Like the hair, the nails are also outgrowths of keratin, and like hair they also develop air spaces in them which turns them white, and this is seen especially in those who are short of the mineral zinc. The nail bed, which is just behind the cuticle, is where the nails form so any trauma here is likely to leave a legacy for some three months while the nail grows out. It is seen as either a midline groove in those who pick their cuticle, or as a transverse line (Beau's line) in those whose nails temporarily stop growing during a severe illness. More severe damage results in the nail

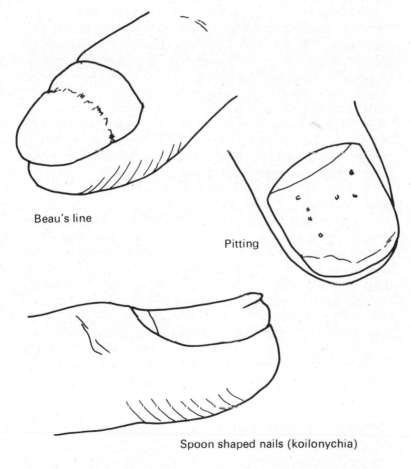

Beau's line

Pitting

Spoon shaped nails (koilonychia)

FIGURE 4.1   *Examples of nail pathology*

becoming greatly thickened and curved, seen especially in the toes of jockeys and stable lads.

Discolouration of the nail is common, especially in those who enjoy gardening, when strands of fungi may become lodged in the cracks and gradually turn the nail yellow, green or brown, pervading the keratin and separating it from its bed. A similar fungal disorder affects those who immerse their hands in water frequently and causes inflammation of the cuticle (*paronychia*) which becomes red and soggy. In cases of liver and kidney disease. where there is a reduction in the serum proteins, the nail may become very pale or even quite white, and sometimes this is confined to the half moons at the proximal aspect of the nail.

Distortion of the nail is seen particularlly in severe iron deficiency when there is a *spoon-shaped*, dry, brittle nail which cracks easily ('koilonychia'), and this also occurs in myxoedema. Psoriasis leads to the familiar pitting of nails by involving the nail bed, and sometimes even lifts the nail off its bed altogether and discolours it.

SKIN TUMOURS

Lumps appearing on the skin may arise from one or more of a number of structures and this has given rise to a variety of descriptive terms such as 'naevus', 'mole', 'wart', etc which are not always accurate and do not always distinguish between benign and malignant lesions.

Benign Tumours

At birth almost all babies have some form of skin blemish ranging from the common 'stork mark' of dilated capillaries on the neck or the bridge of the nose, to the *'strawberry mark'* or cavernous naevus which is sometimes quite large but almost always disappears by the fifth year of life. Occasionally babies are born with an extensive capillary naevus with a network of dilated capillaries called the *port wine stain* which persists. Incidentally the word 'naevus' actually means 'mole' in Latin but has come to refer to tumours involving the vessels.

Moles are collections of melanocytes, the pigment containing cells of the skin, which usually develop in the course of a lifetime, sometimes in large numbers. If one is present at birth then it tends to cause distortion of the hair follicles in that area resulting in a tuft of coarse hair surmounting it. Moles take many shapes and sizes and are often multiple, ranging from light pink to dark brown. Only very rarely to they become malignant (see below) and this is more likely where they are large or deeply pigmented. In old age a rather peculiar type of benign but very warty-looking mole may develop, particularly on the temples, neck or trunk. These are known as *seborrheic* or *senile warts* and have a greasy appearance, sometimes reaching an inch or more in diameter.

Sebaceous cysts, or 'wens' as they are sometimes called, are cysts of the sebaceous glands attached to the hair follicles and are thus found principally on the scalp where they grow to look like a round grape-size swelling. They seldom become inflamed or cause any problems other than cosmetic ones. Similar round swellings called *lipomas* appear on the body, usually the areas where there is subcutaneous fat in some abundance such as the hips, trunk, thighs or upper arms. They are solid benign tumours of fat, distinguishable by being soft, painless and freely mobile when palated.

Malignant Tumours

There are only three skin cancers which are seen with any degree of frequency, and they are all becoming more frequent, mainly because we expose ourselves more and more to the sun.

Melanomas in particular are five times as common as they were forty years ago and half of them arise in normal skin, the rest in moles. The first evidence is either a darkening in colour, itching, bleeding, spreading or ulceration and any of these symptoms should be viewed with suspicion as there is a risk of distant metatases occurring. Once the tumour has spread to the local lymph nodes only about one third of patients survive more than five years, especially if the original lesion is on the upper half of the body.

Epitheliomas or *squamous cell carcinomas* tend to arise on parts of the skin damaged by ultraviolet light, so they are common in places like Australia and South Africa among the white population and are usually seen on the face, ears, hands etc. They look like a small papule to begin with but soon ulcerate and bleed, growing more slowly than a melanoma and metastasizing later.

A somewhat similar appearance of ulceration on the face is seen in the *basal cell carcimoma*, more familiar as the *rodent ulcer*. Its name derives from its habit of destroying any tissue it meets locally and if left will grow extremely large, but it does not metastasize to other parts of the body. It is recognisable by its site on the cheek, nose or lip and its raised, rolled edge with a raw centre which bleeds periodically and then scabs over. It is seen mostly in the elderly, especially if they have been exposed to the sun for many years.

CHAPTER FIVE

BONE:
DISORDERS OF
SUPPORT

Bone is a living tissue and as such is constantly changing, in the sense that its constituents are continually being deposited and removed. Bone consists of an interwoven meshwork of collagen fibres known as a matrix, bound together and hardened by the mineral calcium phosphate, with small traces of magnesium and fluoride which are also necessary to maintain bone health. The regulation of the living matrix of the bone is performed by three different types of cells which create, preserve and destroy it and are known as *osteoblasts, osteocytes* and *osteoclasts* respectively.

Osteoblasts are continually building up new bone and are therefore especially active in childhood when the bones are growing. They leave behind them the osteocytes which are the stable bone cells that act as 'caretakers', but also detect if any fractures or undue stresses take place, when they summon the osteoblasts back to undertake repairs. Osteoclasts are responsible for removing unwanted bone and become especially active if there are insufficient oestrogens to inhibit them, or if they are stimulated by an excess of cortisone in the blood, as we shall see later. Obviously these three have to operate in an integrated manner if health is to be maintained, and disease of bone is usually due either to an ambalance in their conduct or, less commonly, to abnormalities of hormone production.

The rate at which minerals are deposited and removed from the matrix is undertaken by two hormones, *parathormone* and *calcitonin*. The first of these, parathyroid hormone, dissolves calcium from the bones in order to maintain sufficient calcium in the blood, since this must be kept at a constant level even at the expense of the bones. The other calcium controlling hormone, calcitonin, has the opposite effect and reduces the amount of calcium leached from the bones if the level in the blood gets too high.

Vitamin D also plays a vital part in the metabolism of calcium by increasing the ability of the gut to absorb calcium in the diet, and by aiding the mineralisation of bones. Vitamin D is present in animal fats and dairy products, but can also be synthesized by the action of sunlight on the skin.

DEVELOPMENT OF BONE

The skeleton begins to form in the intra-uterine period, and is initially constructed of cartilage alone. By about the sixth month mineralisation begins and calcium is taken from the mother's blood for this purpose, and if necessary from her bones as well. Hence it is important for pregnant mothers to maintain an adequate diet of calcium, of which milk is a very good source.

As the child begins to grow the bones elongate, the growth point being at a band across the end of the bone just below the joint, known as the epiphysis. It is at the epiphysis that large quantities of osteoblasts are engaged in producing new bone, which is later hardened by ossification with the deposit of minerals. Occasionally a child will fracture this epiphysis during a fall and if the bone is not accurately realigned then it will form a *slipped epiphysis* and grow crookedly thereafter, so injuries at the ends of bones in childhood should be treated with great care.

Occasionally children suffer from the congenital disease of *achondroplasia*, and are born without any functioning epiphyseal cartilage in the long bones of the body, so their limbs remain short throughout life although the bones of the rest of the skeleton are quite normal.

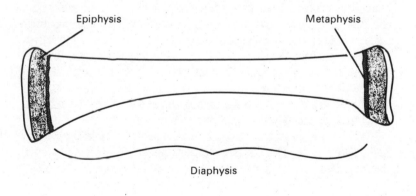

Epiphysis   Metaphysis

Diaphysis

FIGURE 5.1   *Anatomy of a long bone*

At the end of puberty growth of long bones terminates with the fusion of the epiphysis to prevent excessive height, but during the growth period of childhood some epiphyses are vulnerable to minor trauma, particularly the hip, the spine, the carpals of the wrist and the metatarsals in the feet. If the blood supply is temporarily suspended, e.g. from injury, the growing bone will soften for a while and may distort from pressure before hardening again. This process is named *osteochondritis* (juvenilis) and leads to local pain in the area affected, with stiffness if a joint is involved (usually the hip). Provided the softened bone is protected there is no distortion and no later disability but if, in the case of the hip, the child is allowed to walk, then later on osteoarthritis will set in. The different areas of the body where osteochondritis can occur are named after those who first described them, thus:

- *Perthe's disease* affects the hip to cause a limp and pain ('coxalgia').
- *Scheuermann's disease* affects the spine in adolescents and may cause pain and kyphosis.
- *Kienbock's disease* affects the lunate bone of the wrist.
- *Freiburg's disease* affects the head of the metatarsals and may cause pain on walking.

RICKETS AND OSTEOMALACIA

These are essentially two names for similar conditions, rickets being the form which occurs in childhood and osteomalacia that which is seen in adults. Both are caused by a lack of vitamin D, usually because of a combination of poor diet with lack of sunlight. Rickets was seen in the past among impoverished children who grew up in smoky cities and seldom saw the sun, and though now rare in the West is still seen in babies in underdeveloped countries. Since at the time of growth most of the activity of the bone-forming cells is at the epiphyseal line, it is here that any deficiencies in the deposition of minerals, for which vitamin D is responsible, will show up as swelling and softening in the form of *rickets*. These swellings are seen especially at the *wrists* and the *rib cartilages* where they resemble a necklace, the 'rickety rosary'.

Once the epiphyses have fused in adulthood then vitamin D deficiency has a more general effect on the bones, and the skeleton becomes in effect demineralised, a condition called *osteomalacia*. As well as absence of vitamin D, lack of calcium in the blood will also have the effect of demineralising the bones, so osteomalacia may be a result of chronic renal failure losing calcium from the body, or of adult coeliac disease preventing it from being absorbed. The classical cause of vitamin D lack may be seen sometimes in women from the Middle East whose skin is never exposed to the sun, and especially at the time of pregnancy, when the demand is greatest, they may experience general aches and pains in the bones, and great weakness of the muscles (since calcium also plays a large part in enabling muscles to contract). In fact if the blood calcium should descend below a minimal level required by the muscles a form of spasm called *tetany* results (not to be confused with the infectious disease tetanus).

CURVATURE OF THE SPINE

The normal spine possesses a gentle curve convex at the shoulders and concave at the waist, and these are described as a dorsal *kyphosis* (Gr = stooping) and a lumbar *lordosis* (L = to praise) respectively. However, the normal curves may become exaggerated as in osteoporosis or simply from a bad posture. Another type of abnormal curvature is when there is a sideways deviation or *scoliosis* (Gr = crooked), and this is seen in some teenagers, especially girls, as the spine develops. It is sometimes due to weakness of the muscles on one side as in polio, but more often there is no obvious cause.

OSTEOPOROSIS

This is a much more common condition than osteomalacia (although the two are often confused). It is a situation whereby the bones become less dense, but retain their proportions of matrix and minerals alike, so it is not caused by a lack of calcium alone. Our bones reach a peak in their density at around the age of 35, and thereafter tend to gradually lighten with age. Osteoporosis is said to have occurred if the bones become so weak that they either fracture or crumble, and is very commonly seen in women, who begin to lose bone mass after the menopause. About one woman in four develops an accelerated rate of loss such that by her seventies the bones will tend to fracture very easily in the event of a fall.

The increase in the activity of osteoclasts in women is due to a fall in the circulating oestrogens which happens naturally around the time of the menopause and may begin rather before. Men also occasionally develop osteoporosis, but in their case it is because there is a great reduction in the formation of new bone rather than because of the increase in bone absorption, and is unrelated to hormone imbalance.

Why is it, then, that some women develop severe bone failure as they grow older, yet some are immune from the effects? The answer is partly an inherited one, since the greater the mass of bone in youth, the longer it will take for the onset of osteoporosis. Similarly if the menopause is delayed or the woman has had many children (which raises the level of oestrogens). It is interesting that women who develop primary osteo-arthritis of the fingers (see Chap 6) have relatively dense bone and less chance of fractures.

On the other hand certain factors increase the risk of developing osteoporosis, including smoking, poor diet, hyperthyroidism, treatment with cortisone and lack of exercise. The latter is necessary in order to stress the bones and stimulate the activity of osteoblasts. Anorexia nervosa in earlier life is also a cause of later bone problems, as is malabsorption from coeliac disease. It is in these women that *hormone replacement therapy* (HRT) is offered as a means of preventing osteoporosis, but this must be taken within a few years of the menopause in order to prevent the loss of bone, for once lost there is no possibility of replacement. HRT will, of course, mean the continuation of menstruation, and this may be a nuisance. It is given as a combination of oestrogen and progesterone in small doses, the progesterone being included to prevent excessive growth of the endometrium of the womb which might otherwise become malignant. At one time there was thought to be an increased risk of breast cancer, but recent studies have shown that this is not the case. Because

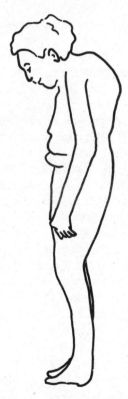

FIGURE 5.2   *Typical posture of osteoporosis*

older people are less able to absorb calcium from their food, supplementary calcium and vitamin D should also be given.

Osteoporosis leads to symptoms in various bones, usually as a fracture. An elderly person is more likely to fall and the commonest bones to break are those of the wrist and of the hip. The former, known as a Colle's fracture, is not too serious and will usually only require a splint for a few weeks, but a fracture through the neck of the femur can often create problems and may even necessitate a hip replacement. Moreover it can create a lack of independence thereafter, and there is a considerable risk of pneumonia developing. The other bones which are liable to fracture are the vertebrae, which become compressed – a *compression fracture*. This usually happens at the front of the body of the vertebra, so the spine becomes bowed forward and a kyphotic posture is assumed – the 'dowager's hump'. The compression of the abdominal contents may lead to urinary incontinence or a hiatus hernia, and if the collapse happens suddenly then there will usually be a severe pain in the back radiating around to the chest or abdomen.

PAGET'S DISEASE

Once again, this is a disorder of the normal balance between creation and destruction of bone, but in this case it is the osteoblasts which err on the side of creating more bone than is needed and in a somewhat irregular fashion, so that large cavities are left. These spaces are filled with very vascular fibrous tissue, and occupied by such a large volume of blood that eventually the patient may go into heart failure in the effort to maintain such a large circulation. The bones enlarge and distort as they expand, and the first part to be noticed may be the cranium when a larger hat is required. The long bones of the body also become bowed, thickened and irregular, hence the alternative name of 'osteitis deformans' for this condition, and the spine develops a kyphosis.

Paget's disease is restricted to people over the age of 50 and is mild in most of them, perhaps even passing unnoticed unless the skull is X-rayed when increased density of bone is seen. In others it may give rise to pain and headaches from stretching of the periosteum, the pain being usually worse at night. In a small minority, about 1%, the osteoblasts get completely out of hand and become malignant after a few years.

CHAPTER SIX

JOINTS: DISORDERS OF STABILITY

*T*he terms 'arthritis' and 'rheumatism' are often used rather loosely to describe pains which are generally worse from movement, but strictly speaking the word 'arthritis' refers to pain coming from a joint, while 'rheumatism' means any ache or pain which moves about the body and therefore may emanate from muscles, tendons or ligaments. There are many diseases in which arthritis is part of the picture, but only about half a dozen or so are seen with any frequency.

Pain in a joint arises from the surfaces lining it, the cartilage or the synovium, and it is the latter which when inflamed will exude fluid into the joint and make it swell – an *effusion*. The cartilaginous surface of the joint is essentially for absorbing shocks to the bone and so has to withstand huge stresses on occasions. For example the knee joint has a surface area of approximately four square inches and transmits half of the weight of a 200 lb body, a pressure of about 25 lb/sq inch which is equal to that in a car tyre. On walking that pressure is doubled and on running quadrupled, so any excess weight that has to be carried puts it under great stress.

OSTEOARTHRITIS

The cartilage which covers and cushions the ends of bones within the joints may begin to wear out in some people, especially (but not necessarily) in the joints which bear the most weight. This process of wear in a joint is hastened if either the stress is excessive – often because the person is overweight, or if it is applied at a slight angle and not through the centre of the joint, as may happen after a fracture, if the posture is poor, or where the joint is made unstable by some other form of arthritis such as rheumatoid arthritis. This process of physical wearing out or 'eburnation' of the cartilage is the basis of osteoarthritis, and as the cartilage is ground away the bone cells beneath frantically try to repair the damage by proliferating and mineralising the bone, only to have it constantly cracked. Synovial fluid is squeezed into these cracked areas which develop tiny cysts called 'geodes' and this further weakens the bone. The only area where the proliferating bone is not being subjected to this pounding is at the very edges of the joint, and here irregular swellings called *osteophytes* grow, seen most clearly as *Heberden's nodes* in the fingers.

Primary osteoarthritis is the name given to the type occurring on account of age, and is usually seen in the *knees* and *hands*, also in the *hips*, *spine* and less commonly in the shoulders. As a rule only a few joints are affected, and the age when they start to cause symptoms is from around the fifties onwards. Women are rather more affected than men by OA, and about one in five develop symptoms of it at some time.

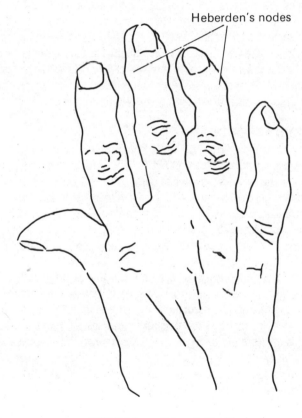

Heberden's nodes

FIGURE 6.1   *Osteoarthritis of the hand*

When the intricate joints of the spine, particularly the facet joints, are afflicted by these ailments, the term *spondylosis* is used (Gr.

69

spondylos = vertebra), and is the source of much backache in later life. Moreover, the osteophytes which develop in the neck have the habit of pressing on the vertebral arteries which run up inside the cervical vertebral bodies to supply the posterior parts of the cortex. This may lead to neurological symptoms such as dizziness and loss of vision when the head is turned in a certain direction.

Not all joints affected by OA are painful, and it is not uncommon to see the hands painlessly involved, especially the joints indicated in diagram 6.1. If the carpometaphalangeal (CMP) joint at the base of the thumb is involved, however, then this is likely to be painful and quite incapacitating as it affects any activity involving gripping. Pain is also a common feature of OA of the hip, being worse on sudden movement especially going upstairs, and sometimes radiating down the thigh to the knee. If the knee is affected then it is likely to cause pain on walking over uneven ground or on descending the stairs. In all cases the pain is generally worse in cold, damp weather and remains constant during exercise, unlike that of rheumatoid arthritis which usually improves with movement.

RHEUMATOID ARTHRITIS
The disease gets its name from the word 'rheuma', meaning a stream of morbid humours which were considered to flow through the body, and which refers to the widespread flu-like symptoms with aches and pains which are often the earliest indicators of the disease. It is not only the joints which are affected in RA, and the term 'rheumatoid disease' is perhaps more appropriate to describe what is effectively a disorder of connective tissue in the joints, vessels, skin, lungs, eyes and lymphoid tissue.

There are many theories as to the origin of the condition, none of which are totally convincing, and they include infection, autoimmunity, genetic, food sensitivity and psychological. What has been established, however, is that in about 90% of cases an abnormal protein called *rheumatoid factor* is present in the blood. This is known to be an antibody against an antibody – the body appears to have seized one of its small IgG antibodies and made a much larger IgM antibody against it, and this larger antibody then goes on to attack the synovial membrane of the joints and other tissues. However, why this process should suddenly take place in about one person in 50 between the ages of 30–50 is very mysterious. One theory is that the proteins within the joints become damaged by infection or some other means and that this then alters their antigenic structure, making them no longer recognisable to the body which starts to make antibodies against them – an auto-immune disease.

The first signs of something amiss are often insidious and may include a fever, weakness and depression, weight loss or progressive morning stiffness of the hands, feet or knees. Occasionally the onset is sudden and dramatic with only one joint initially involved – a *monoarthritis* as opposed to the ensuing *polyarthritis*. The synovial membranes inflame and secrete fluid into the joint which swells up and becomes extremely tender and stiff during the acute phase. Later the synovium proliferates and thickens (in contrast to OA) to produce what is called a *pannus* (L. = cloak), and if the joint is not mobilised then there is a risk that the two synovial membranes will fuse and produce an immobile, useless joint. It is this pannus which causes the persistent pain, stiffness and limited range of movement in affected joints (and which is removed in the operation of synovectomy).

However the condition starts, it is likely to progress to a polyarthritis, where several joints are affected though not necessarily severely, and these are commonly the hands which are a prime target. They develop characteristic swelling of the knuckles which deviate towards the ulna, and of the proximal interphalangeal joints (finger joints nearest the knuckles) which develop a spindle shape and sometimes the characteristic *swan neck deformity* of the fingers or the *Z deformity* of the thumbs (see figure 6.2).

As well as the hands, any synovial joint may be involved, and especially the wrists, elbows, shoulders, knees and feet, less commonly the hips, ankles and spine. The same joints are involved in the feet as in the hands, and give the sensation of walking on pebbles in bare feet as the metatarsals are unstable, requiring special shoes. If the knees are involved there is wasting of the quadriceps muscle of the thigh and a *Baker's cyst* may emerge from the rear of the joint as a soft swelling of the weak point of the joint capsule, and possibly even rupture into the muscles of the calf to simulate a deep vein thrombosis.

Involvement of the cervical spine is not infrequent and gives rise to pain in the upper part of the neck. Where the atlanto-axial joint is involved there is the possibility of dangerous instability of the odontoid peg where it passes through the atlas and may subluxate (partially dislocate) to press on the spinal cord, so patients complaining of pains running up to the scalp should be treated with circumspection.

Non Articular Manifestations
Many other body systems may be involved in RA, some of which are rare and will not be discussed. One of the more common is the *subcutaneous nodule* seen on the bony prominences of the elbows, shoulders and knees

or the tendons of the wrists and feet. They are hard, painless swellings of degenerating connective tissue, up to 1″ in diameter, formed in response to leakage of the rheumatoid factor from damaged vessels. Another common concomitant of RA is *anaemia* which arises because the marrow is inhibited from taking up iron (although there is no shortage in the body), and this and the thinning of the skin which occurs gives the patient a pale, waxy complexion. Some cases of anaemia are made worse by gastric bleeding from aspirin and other drugs taken for the arthritis.

Spindle-shaped swelling

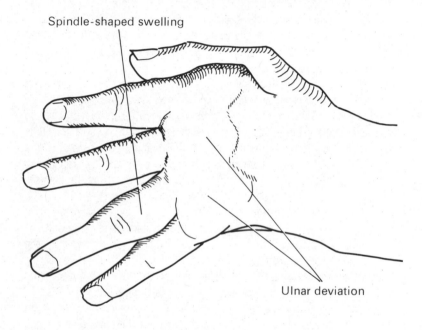

Ulnar deviation

FIGURE 6.2   *Advanced rheumatoid arthritis of the hand*

The *lymph nodes* are sometimes enlarged, often in the neighbour-hood of a badly affected joint, and this is especially seen in children who have a slightly different and rare form of RA known as *Still's disease* which includes general swelling of the lymph glands and spleen.

Another fairly frequent consequence, affecting about 15% of those with RA, is the drying up of the secretions of the salivary and the tear glands, a condition termed *Sjogren's syndrome*. This leads to difficulty with swallowing and sore, inflamed eyes especially around the whites of the eye (episcleritis).

The appearance of breathlessness in especially men with RA may indicate that the pleura has become involved and has reacted by forming a *pleural effusion*. Women are more likely to notice compression of the median nerve in the wrist and feel tingling sensations in the hands – the *carpal tunnel syndrome*.

GOUT

Despite its music hall image gout is one of the most painful conditions known to man (women are generally immune until after the menopause), and was well described by Hippocrates. Pitt the Elder suffered severely from gout all his life and had to be wheeled about in a specially constructed chair, which has perhaps encouraged the view that it is a disease of retired colonels brought on by high living. In fact the average sufferer of gout is a young man in his 20s or 30s who develops intermittent pains at the base of his big toe which are easily ascribed to strain or injury until they flare up and the joint becomes hot, red and swollen ('podagra').

The problem is one of uric acid crystals forming in the joints and other places, usually because the amount in the blood is excessive. Uric acid is made from DNA and RNA, the constituents of the nuclei of the cells, and these are broken down in the liver and passed to the blood for excretion. The amount which the kidney can excrete is limited, and if this level is exceeded then the 'pool' builds up and some of it crystallises in the joints, the kidney or the cartilage (the latter known as *tophi*). The preferred joint is the *metatarsophalangeal* (MTP) joint of the toe (see figure 6.3), perhaps because it is the lowest, or the coldest, in the body. Sometimes other joints in the body become affected, particularly the knee and elbow, and develop excruciating pain on movement or touch.

If uric acid crystals are formed very rapidly by the body then they may occur as *stones in the kidney* or even crystallise in the tubules and lead to renal failure, although this is rare. Tophaceous deposits are seen in longstanding gouty subjects and occupy the pinna of the ears and the tendons of the arms, where they may eventually ulcerate and exude chalky material (L. tofus = rock).

Gout tends to run in families, and after a first attack there may be no further ones, or they may be few and far between. It is worth avoiding rich foods such as red meat and dairy products as far as possible, as this is often successful in preventing further attacks. Such attacks may sometimes be precipitated by diuretics, when the fluid level of the body drops and effectively increases the uric acid in the blood, or if the body is breaking down an excessive number of cells as in leukaemia or psoriasis.

Uric acid is not the only substance to crystallise out in the joints, however, and elderly people are sometimes liable to what is known as 'pseudogout'. In this much less painful condition the large joints, especially the knees, are affected and the mineral in question is a calcium salt, calcium pyrophosphate. The joints do become severely disrupted, however, and this may later lead to osteoarthritis.

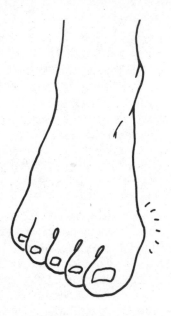

FIGURE 6.3   *Gout, showing the joint most frequently affected*

ANKYLOSING SPONDYLITIS

The joint pathology we have been looking at so far is confined to the synovial joints, those containing fluid and designed for greater movement than the more limited cartilaginous joints. These are seen in the spine linking the vertebrae, and in the ribs and sternum where large movements are not needed, so the elasticity of the cartilage will suffice. Unfortunately these joints too are not without their problems on occasions, and are liable to calcification and even eventually ossification when the cartilage is replaced by bony tissue. If that happens then no movement is possible and the joint is said to be *ankylosed.*

Since the word for spinal arthritis is 'spondylitis', the disease of *ankylosing spondylitis* indicates stiffening of the spine, and that is the main long term effect of the condition. It comes about by gradual ossification of the intervertebral discs, but the earliest signs are in either the *sacro iliac joints* or in the periphery of the body where the cartilaginous tendons are inserted into the bone (the 'entheses'). The favoured entheses where calcification takes place are the sole of the foot in the plantar fascia (*plantar fasciitis*), the Achilles tendon (tendinitis), the hip bones and the shoulder girdle, and these will all be tender on palpation. The classic site for AS, however, is the sacroiliac joint which becomes progressively fused and stiff and usually heralds the onset of the condition.

The story is one of stiffness and aching in the lower back on waking in the mornings, usually in a young man, and the pain eases with movement only to recur on sitting for long periods during the day. There is also a feeling of progressive, inexplicable weakness and fatigue in some, who may be suspected of malingering until the other symptoms make themselves known. Gradually the flexibility of the spine is lost, especially if mobilisation exercises are not encouraged, and much damage is done by resting. This leads to rapid spinal rigidity with swollen, calcified discs – the *bamboo spine* – so called because of its similarity on X-ray to a stem of bamboo. Men are far more likely than women to be affected by this disease, often in their adolescence or early adult life, and some of them will go on to develop complications. These include an *iritis* and take the form of a sore, red eye, or less commonly damage to the aorta and the aortic valve.

TABLE 6.1	Possible causes of arthritis
Condition	**Pointers**
Osteoarthritis	Single joint, worse on use
Rheumatoid arthritis	General debility, fever, joint pattern
Gout	Usually toe, very tender
Ankylosing spondylitis	Worse mornings, young men
Reiter's disease	Urethritis, conjunctivitis
Ulcerative colitis	Bloodstained diarrhoea
Crohn's disease	Abdominal pain, diarrhoea
Lupus erythematosis	Skin rash, kidney problems
Rheumatic fever	Pyrexia, rash, heart murmur, sore throat
Sarcoidosis	Wheeze, cough
Psoriasis	Skin rash, nail pitting
Septic arthritis	Extreme tenderness, fever
Henoch-Schonlein purpura	Children, abdo pain, bloody diarrhoea, rash
Behcet's syndrome	Oral & genital ulceration, iritis

REITER'S SYNDROME

Reiter originally described a triad of symptoms, composed of arthritis, urethritis and either iritis or conjunctivitis. These were observed to follow an infection 3–4 weeks previously, usually a venereal infection with a urethral discharge but sometimes an acute bowel infection with diarrhoea. It now seems clear that both Reiter's disease and ankylosing spondylitis are forms of 'reactive arthritis' which are started by an environmental trigger. In the case of AS the trigger factor is unknown, but in Reiter's disease it is either a chlamydia, shigella (dysentery), salmonella or campylobacter infection, although the first of these is the most common.

Both Reiter's disease and AS are linked to the presence of the antigen HLA B27 on the cells of the body (see Chap 2), and both this and the trigger factor have to be present for the disease to occur. There are many conditions where this is a factor, which is why several conditions such as psoriasis, Crohn's disease and ulcerative colitis exhibit arthritis as one of the possible symptoms. Reiter's disease affects the large synovial joints and sometimes cartilaginous joints as well, and in some people skin rashes may also occur.

DRUGS AND ARTHRITIS

For many years aspirin, originally distilled from willow bark in 1837, was the favoured drug for use in arthritis, though the method by which it operated has remained a mystery until recently. It now appears that it has an effect on the group of substances known as the *prostaglandins*, because they were originally found in high concentration in seminal fluid in the prostate gland. There are numerous different prostaglandins in a variety of human tissues, each having a particular effect. For instance in women certain prostaglandins stimulate ovulation and have a powerful influence on the uterus so are used to induce labour or terminate a pregnancy. Another has an effect on the brain, where it causes a rise in temperature in response to bacterial pyrogenic toxins by acting on the temperature centre. Yet another is produced by platelets to increase their stickiness and promote clotting.

The effect of aspirin is to inhibit many of these functions of prostaglandins, so it prevents a rise in temperature and inhibits the action of platelets which is often useful where there is a tendency to thrombosis. Its best-known function, though, is as an *analgesic*, that is to say a pain-killer. Because prostaglandins sensitise the nerve endings to painful stimuli, by blocking these some relief is obtained, and this is particularly useful in mild arthritis, especially if there is an accompanying fever such as rheumatic fever. When its mode of action was discovered, a search was made for other anti-prostaglandin drugs in the hope that these would have fewer of the side effects, the most notable being gastric bleeding and ulceration.

It was known that cortisone (see chapter 16) was a strong anti-inflammatory drug, but operated in a very different manner and caused numerous unwanted effects. However, drugs analogous to aspirin were soon discovered, of varying potency and side-effects, and these were given the name 'non-steroidal anti-inflammatory drugs' or NSAIDS. The original preparation, butazolidin or 'bute' for short, was both very powerful and very toxic to the blood, so has now been discontinued except for occasional hospital use. The most commonly-used NSAIDS (with the brand names in brackets) are given in the table below.

Drug	Comments
Naproxen (Naprosyn)*	Safe, free of most side-effects
Ibuprofen (Brufen)*	Safe, weak anti-inflammatory
Benorylate (Benoral)*	Mixture of aspirin & paracetamol esters
Ketoprofen (Orudis)	Used for dysmenorrhoea
Piroxicam (Feldene)	Longer action, more gastric effects
Azapropazone (Rheumox)	Possible photosensitivity
Diclofenac (Voltarol)	Stronger analgesic
Indomethacin (Indocid)	Strong, but more side-effects

List of NSAIDS in common use (* indicates over-the-counter availability)

Today NSAIDS are among the most widely prescribed drugs, for they act against pain, inflammation and thrombosis which are three of the commonest symptoms. The market is therefore fiercely contested and well over fifty preparations are available, but people will usually react differently to a drug, so often several are tried in sequence. The unwanted effects can be grouped into four categories, the first being that of gastric effects similar to aspirin but not usually as severe. Another possible effect, which varies from drug to drug, is hypersensitivity, which takes the form of asthma, urticaria or a rash and is uncommon. If the drug is taken excessively, then it is likely to affect the middle ear and cause tinnitus, deafness, vertigo or a headache. Finally most NSAIDS will encourage the retention of fluid in someone who is predisposed to it, usually an older person.

Can one stop taking these drugs without harm? The answer is yes, but of course there may be some pain for a while until some other form of treatment takes effect. If aspirin has been given for the prevention of a stroke or heart attack, rather than for pain, then there is a very small risk that one could be induced.

CHAPTER SEVEN

MUSCLES & TENDONS: DISORDERS OF MOVEMENT

*T*he muscles of the body form a system of levers which operate the joints, and in most cases span the joint either alone or with the aid of a tendon. Trauma or overuse can easily damage either the muscle or its tendon, and in the case of the latter this is particularly serious as it is much less vascular and takes far longer to heal. A pulled muscle indicates that some of the fibres are torn, usually on account of violent or unaccustomed exercise, and this is much more likely in cold, tight muscles which have not been warmed up gradually. It is thus very important to do warm-up exercises before sport, especially in the older age-groups whose muscles are more susceptible to damage. *Cramp* is another way in which muscles protest at overuse or insufficient blood. Sometimes pain arises spontaneously in a muscle which goes into spasm in certain areas which become tender and swollen as *fibrositis*, and this is liable to happen especially in the large muscles of the lower back and is termed *lumbago*.

Ligaments, which connect bone to bone and stabilise the joints, are liable to *sprain* if excess force is used on a joint, and although they are elastic, if the sprain is severe the ligament is left stretched and swollen. The immediate treatment of a sprain is to apply a cold compress with a crepe bandage and rest the limb by elevating it to reduce swelling. If the joint itself is damaged then the muscles which operate it will tend to atrophy unless exercised, and rehabilitation plays a large part in such injuries. Actual paralysis or weakness of a muscle is almost always due to neurological problems, apart from the rare congenital muscular dystrophies and myasthenia gravis.

Apart from accidents and disease, there are two ways in which muscles and tendons get damaged, and these reflect our increasingly competitive world – *sports injuries* and *repetitive strain injuries*. Both of these have become much more prevalent of late, and their recognition and prevention is now an important part of health care.

Because of the complex interaction of muscles, tendons, joints and ligaments it is preferable to depart for a while from the systems approach and look at the soft tissues in various areas of the body individually.

THE SPINE

Unlike the limbs, the spine is not a lever. This may appear to be stating the obvious but many of the problems which the back incurs arise from using it as if it were. Nature designed the spine for both support and flexibility, and did so by wedging it in the pelvis at the sacroiliac joints and then 'guying' it with muscles. It is when these muscles are not properly used or become slack that the intervertebral joints and discs develop displacements which may lead to pressure on the nerve roots as they emerge from the spine. If they are compressed then the person experiences referred pain in the area supplied by the nerve and may additionally notice weakness of the muscles. The nerves supplying the arm and the leg are most likely to be affected and the pain is then termed *brachial neuralgia* or *sciatica* respectively.

THE SHOULDER

Nature had to compromise on the stability of the shoulder joint in order to

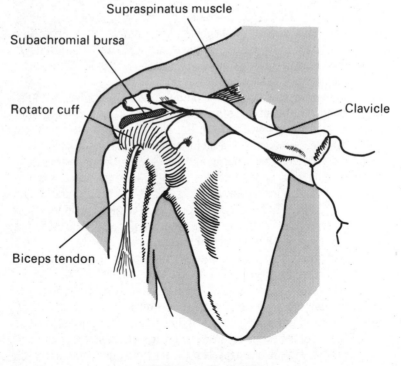

Supraspinatus muscle

Subachromial bursa

Rotator cuff

Clavicle

Biceps tendon

FIGURE 7.1   *The shoulder*

maximise the range of movements available to the arm, and did so by making the socket (glenoid cavity) in the scapula rather shallow, which allows the shoulder to dislocate downwards very easily. Once this happens, the contour of the joint immediately appears misshapen, but even after the humerus has been returned to the glenoid cavity of the scapula, the ligaments are so badly stretched that recurrent dislocations are common at the slightest provocation.

Compensation for the lack of bony protection to the joint comes in the form of a ring of muscles and ligaments which grip the head of the humerus firmly like a 'lions claw' and form the *rotator cuff*. If this becomes inflamed or damaged then the shoulder sustains pain on the least movement in any direction – the *frozen shoulder*. This may follow an injury or in older people come on spontaneously, and as the pain gradually lessens so the stiffness increases and may limit movements for many months unless adequate therapy is forthcoming.

If, however, inflammation is limited to one of the muscles or tendons

TABLE 7.1 Possible causes of backache	
Condition	Pointers
Muscular strain	History, tender muscles
Ligamentous strain	History, painful movements
Facet joint disturbance	Lack of symmetry, local pain
Postural	Examination, work history
Prolapsed disc	Referred pain, worse on leg raising
Obesity	Obvious
Pregnancy	Obvious
Osteoarthritis	Other joints affected
Osteoporosis	Age, sudden onset, localised
Ankylosing spondylitis	Worse mornings
Metastasis	Usually from breast, lung, prostate, kidney
Polymyalgia rheumatica	Elderly, headaches, muscle weakness
Tuberculosis	Rare, may be weight loss
Paget's disease	Large skull, distorted bones
Myeloma	Elderly, proteinuria
Referred CVS	Myocardial infarct, aortic aneurysm
Referred lungs	Pleurisy, pulmonary infarction
Referred abdo	Pancreatic cancer, urinary infection
Referred pelvis	Salpingitis, endometriosis, dysmenorrhoea
Referred skin	Herpes zoster

running over the joint then only the movements initiated by that muscle are painful. Thus *biceps tendenitis* will cause pain over the front of the joint on lifting, as the biceps tendon runs in this area and is commonly strained in weightlifters, rowers and golfers. Beneath the deltoid muscle is a bursa which protects the muscle when the arms are raised sideways, and this sometimes becomes inflamed as a *bursitis* if overuse occurs. A similar bursa exists a little higher, the 'subachromial bursa', and both are commonly inflamed in tennis and gymnastics. There is a painful arc when the arm is raised, between 45 and 90 degrees, after which it becomes pain-free.

The shoulder may also be affected by any condition damaging the sympathetic nerve supply of the region, particularly a stroke, myocardial infarction or cervical spondylosis. This can reduce the blood flow to the shoulder and hand together, and the two become cold and atrophied – the *shoulder-hand syndrome*.

THE ELBOW

This is a hinge joint between the ulna and the humerus, and also contains a pivot between the head of the radius and the ulna to allow the forearm to pronate and supinate. The annular ligament retaining the head of the radius in position is relatively weak in young children, so that a sudden jerk on their hand may pull the radial head through the ligament (*pulled elbow*). The hand will then be held pronated across the body until the radius is replaced by firm pressure with supination which 'screws' the head back into place.

The olecranon process at the back of the elbow is protected by a

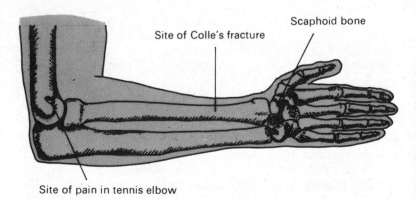

Scaphoid bone

Site of Colle's fracture

Site of pain in tennis elbow

FIGURE 7.2   *The elbow and hand*

bursa which may become inflamed in someone who spends a lot of time leaning on their elbows, such as a student. This swells up into an *olecranon bursitis* the size of a golf ball for a few days, but usually disappears with rest. Just above the capitulum of the humerus (see figure) is the origin of the forearm abductor muscles which operate the wrist. You can feel this on yourself by folding your arms, when the little finger of your right hand will lie over the point, and if you now extend the fingers of your left hand you will feel the tendon contract. It is tendinitis at this exact location, caused by overuse of the wrist in hammering, sawing or tennis, which is known as *tennis elbow*. A similar tendinitis on the medial side is called *golfer's* or *javelin thrower's elbow*.

THE WRIST & HAND

Many of the movements in this area are performed by muscles located in the forearms and operating by long tendons which run across the wrist and into the hand. This exposes the joint to sprains and fractures, as well as inflammation of the tendon sheaths (*tenosynovitis*). In the latter condition the synovial sheath covering the tendon becomes inflamed from overuse and swells, pinching the tendon and making it difficult to use as well as painful. If this happens to the tendon supplying the finger flexors, then it may be difficult to straighten the finger after flexion (*trigger finger*). When it occurs in the abductor tendons to the thumb it is sometimes called *de Quervain's syndrome*, and may be a symptom of RA or of too much canoeing (paddler's wrist).

A more common condition is that known as *Dupuytren's contracture*, which is a thickening of the tendons which run across the palm of the hand, especially those supplying the little and ring fingers. This causes painless shortening and consequent flexion of the fingers which weakens the grip. It tends to be a familial complaint, but is also more common in those who have epilepsy or alcoholism.

A fall on the outstretched hand is likely to cause a fracture in the locality, either a *Colle's fracture* of the ulna in the elderly, with its typical 'dinner fork' displacement, or a *scaphoid fracture* in the young, with tenderness in the 'anatomical snuffbox' when it is pinched. Because of the large number of tiny carpal bones in the wrist and the joints between them, swellings of synovial membrane may extrude from the joints in the area and form what are known (inaccurately) as *ganglia*. They are painless and nothing more than unsightly, but it is not recommended that they be ruptured, either by the family bible or anything else.

The anterior aspect of the wrist is covered by a band of fibrous tissue which guides the flexor tendons and the median nerve through the carpal

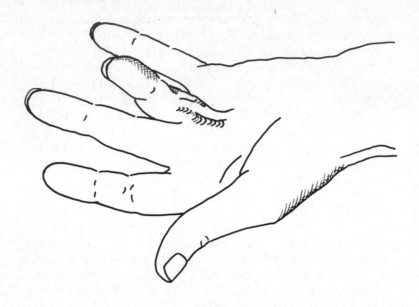

FIGURE 7.3   *Dupuytren's contracture*

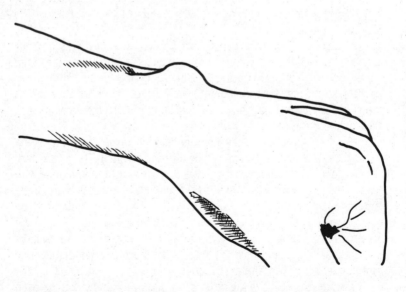

FIGURE 7.4   *Ganglion*

tunnel beneath. If damaged by trauma or arthritis, or if the underlying tissues swell from oedema or myxoedema, the resultant pressure on the nerve will lead to pain, tingling and weakness of the fingers, particularly at night, the well known *carpal tunnel syndrome*. Many individuals with no overt pathology suffer from this condition, particularly at night, and a useful test is gently to extend the wrist which brings on the symptoms.

THE KNEE

This is a hinge joint and somewhat vulnerable as it is unprotected by muscle tissue. Moreover it has to transmit some truly enormous strains through the tendons which cross it, and relies heavily on ligaments to keep the joint surfaces in place. As well as the articular cartilage common to all synovial joints, the tibial surface possesses two thick pads called menisci, semilunar cartilages which act as additional shock absorbers. These are liable to tear if the knee is flexed to a right angle and then twisted, as happens often in football or mining injuries, when the condyle which protrudes from the femur will grind it into the tibia and tear it. These torn

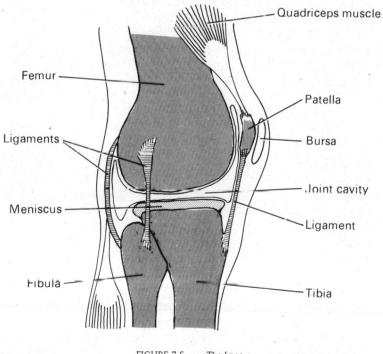

FIGURE 7.5　　*The knee*

menisci will then flap about and jam in the joint when it bends, leading to locking, which is the main symptom of a 'torn cartilage'. If the stresses to the knee come from the side or the front, then the supporting ligaments which join the bones are liable to be stretched and torn, leading to local tenderness and swelling of the joint. This *effusion* into the joint happens because some of the ligaments actually run inside the joint capsule.

The most important structures supporting the knee, however, are the muscles, especially the large *quadriceps* muscle which is inserted into the tibia at the front, via the patella, and extends the knee. This muscle makes up the bulk of the front of the thigh and if it becomes weakened from damage or disuse then the knee may suddenly give way, as happens particularly in the elderly after they have been ill in bed for some time. It may also occur in teenage girls whose patellar bones may click as they drift laterally across the joint as they walk, because they are too loose. The condition is known as *chondromalacia patellae*, and the remedy is to exercise and tighten the muscles by building them up.

Several conditions are seen which cause pain and swelling around the front of the knee. Several bursae exist here to protect the knee when kneeling, and if one of these gets swollen from pressure or a sudden blow, it is known as *housemaid's knee*. Teenage boys who train very hard in running may develop a painful, tender swelling at the top of the tibia where the quadriceps tendon is inserted into the tibial tuberosity. This is termed *Osgood-Schlatter's disease* and can have quite devastating effects on a sporting career, since the only remedy is to avoid all strenuous activity of the quadriceps for months or even years, but it always settles down at the end of the growth period.

THE ANKLE & FOOT

The ankle is a hinge joint in between a mortice formed by the malleoli of the fibula and tibia, and has little sideways movement except when the toes are pointed. Consequently you are more likely to sprain or even fracture your ankle (*Pott's fracture*) if you walk heavily on your heels rather than your toes on rough ground. The main supports for the ankle are the strong medial and lateral ligaments which are stretched if the foot is forcibly over-adducted or abducted, usually the former. Thus the commonest sprain of the angle is an *inversion sprain* with tenderness and swelling over the lateral ligament, just below the malleolus. If there is tenderness over the lateral malleolus itself then suspect a fracture of the lower end of the fibula, commonly seen after skiing accidents.

At the back of the ankle the Achilles tendon is inserted into the calcaneum, and pain in this area may be due to a tendinitis with inflammation and swelling of the tendon sheath directly behind the ankle. Careful palpation will usually elicit *crepitus*, a slight grating sensation on movement, and this usually occurs from overuse. On occasions the tendon may even rupture during sudden exertion and there will be a palpable gap. Sometimes the pain is felt lower down over the back of the calcaneum, at the point of insertion of the tendon where a bursa is located, which signifies a *calcaneal bursitis*, and is often a problem of those who do a lot of road running with inadequate shoes.

At the front of the bottom of the calcaneum, on the sole of the foot, are inserted the plantar muscles via the plantar fascia, which maintain the arch and spring of the foot. The tendon at this point may calcify and produce a painful *plantar fasciitis*, so the patient develops a limp as he cannot bear weight on this area. This happens in those who have overstretched, poorly-developed arches and do a lot of running; it may in some cases be a sign of ankylosing spondylitis or Reiter's syndrome.

The sole of the foot may also give rise to pain further forward, over the heads of the metatarsal bones and therefore called *metatarsalgia*. Again this may be due to running on hard surfaces in inappropriate shoes, as the first metatarsophalangeal (MTP) joint is very susceptible to trauma and easily becomes stiff and immobile so is given the name *hallux rigidus*. Later this may develop into osteoarthritis of the joint and be confused with gout which has a predilection for the same joint but is far more tender. *Stress fractures* are also common in the metatarsal bones and present with forefoot pain and a limp after severe exercise. They are easily missed as the hairline fracture does not show up on an X-ray until callus has formed several days later.

A very common condition of the feet is *hallux valgus* or *hammer toes*, which tend to be constitutional and run in families. The deformity consists of a 'valgus' or abduction of the MTP joint of the big toe or hallux. This usually develops a large bursa over it known as a *bunion* which becomes inflamed and painful. The second and third toes then become hooked over the hallux and are known as 'claw toes', and these gradually subluxate and lead to instability of the foot with the passage of time.

HERNIAS

One of the main functions of the abdominal muscles is to contain the viscera and keep the organs in position. On occasions they either become too weak or have excess pressure exerted on them, and so a gap appears between the fibres allowing the abdominal organs to partially or completely protrude, this protrusion being a *hernia*. The hernial sac is likely to bulge through in places where there is a potential weakness in the

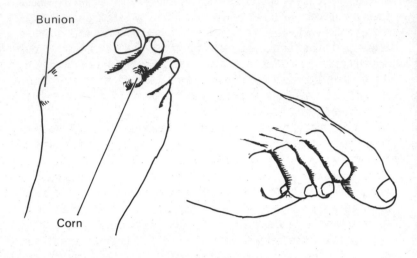

Bunion

Corn

FIGURE 7.6   *A. Hallux valgus, B. Claw toes*

abdominal muscles such as the groin or the diaphragm, often at the site where other structures penetrate the wall. Once the musculature has started to give it is seldom possible to strengthen it by exercises, and the tendency is for the bulge gradually to increase in size as the months go by.

If the hernia goes back inside the abdomen on relaxation or lying down, or can easily be pushed back, then it is said to be *reducible*, but if not then it is *irreducible* and is then at risk of strangulation or obstruction. When a hernia *strangulates* then the blood supply, which accompanies the loop of bowel, is cut off and the bowel begins to die and eventually will become gangrenous if left for longer than about 6–8 hours. *Obstruction* of a hernia means that the contents of the intestine cannot move through it, so there are a series of colicky pains as the pressure builds up. Normally, apart from a heavy, dragging sensation a hernia is painless unless one of these complications occurs, so any pain indicates that intervention is urgently needed.

Inguinal Hernia

This type of hernia is mostly seen in men or boys and is due to the fact that when the testis descends into the scrotum it travels down the inguinal canal in between two layers of muscle in the groin. The entrance to the canal (internal ring) is half an inch above the femoral pulse in the groin,

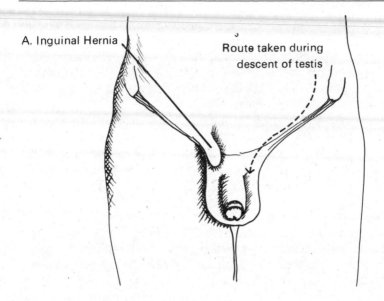

A. Inguinal Hernia

Route taken during
descent of testis

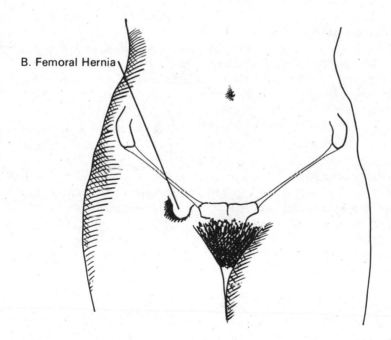

B. Femoral Hernia

FIGURE 7.7   *Hernias in men and women*

and the exit, the external ring, is in the top of the scrotum where it can be palpated, and it is here that the hernia will emerge. Sometimes it can be seen rolling down the inguinal canal when the subject coughs, and a finger over the internal ring will prevent this. This, of course, is the function of a truss, the type of padded belt worn by those who are unfit for an operation to sew up the hernia ('herniorrhaphy').

Occasionally women get inguinal hernias, but in their case the swelling does not go indirectly down the inguinal canal but pushes directly through the weak abdominal wall at the level of the external ring, and this can be proved by the fact that its emergence cannot be prevented by pressure over the internal ring.

Femoral hernia
Because women have a wider pelvis than men the potential space under the inguinal ligament, through which all the vessels and nerves leave for the leg, is much greater, as everything is less packed together. It is down this femoral canal below the inguinal ligament that a hernia may develop, and this can occasionally occur in men in whom the risk of strangulation is high because the aperture is so much smaller.

Umbilical Hernia
These are commonly seen in newborn babies as a soft bulge around the umbilicus, and swell up when the baby cries. They reduce very easily and so there is no risk of strangulation, in fact they only exist because the muscles have not yet developed and almost always disappear within two years. A similar hernia may be seen in women after pregnancy but in this case the swelling is just above the umbilicus and is therefore known as a para-umbilical hernia, and seldom resolves spontaneously.

Incisional Hernia
After a midline abdominal operation or **laparotomy** (Gr. laparos = soft) the muscles are sewn together but never with the original strength so if there is a cough and the intra-abdominal pressure is elevated, or if the wound becomes infected and the tissues break down, the intestines may herniate through and form a large bulge under the skin. This is very unsightly but seldom dangerous and can usually be repaired.

Hiatus Hernia
These are herniations of the stomach through the diaphragm and are covered in Chapter 12.

CHAPTER EIGHT

BLOOD:
DISORDERS OF
TRANSPORT

*B*lood, which circulates in virtually all our tissues, is made up of cells and plasma which each contribute about half the volume. In the event of a serious haemorrhage both, of course, are lost but the body is able to replace the plasma within a matter of hours, since this is composed mainly of water. The cellular component takes a little longer, however, and during this time we are depleted of red and white cells and are slightly anaemic. Because the marrow can produce red cells at the rate of 2.5 million *a second* (if layed edge to edge the daily output would stretch from London to Edinburgh), the anaemia only becomes significant if we continue to lose blood from, say, heavy periods or bleeding piles at a rate faster than the body can produce them. In order for this production line to operate efficiently there must be no shortage of raw materials, and that means protein, vitamin B12, folic acid and, of course, iron.

IRON DEFICIENCY ANAEMIA
The oxygen carrying ability of the red cell is due to the unique properties of haemoglobin, the iron-containing red pigment of which it is composed. This iron has to come from our food and is stored for future use mainly in the liver (which is why this is such a rich natural source). At times of growth and pregnancy these stores may become depleted, and any dietary lack of iron or any inability to absorb it by the small intestine will result in iron deficiency anaemia. For this reason it is a condition mainly of children and women of childbearing age, and about 1 woman in 10 suffers from lack of iron, especially if their menstrual loss is heavy. Delayed weaning in babies may cause iron deficiency as there is very little iron present in milk.

Iron must first be acidified in the stomach before it can go on to be absorbed by the small intestine, so any operation which removes the acid-secreting part of the stomach, such as a *partial gastrectomy* will affect absorption, and so will conditions such as coeliac disease which damages the jejunum.

The most common reason for iron deficiency is simply that there is a continuous loss of blood, either from heavy periods or from somewhere in the gut. So-called *occult bleeding* may feature in peptic ulcer, aspirin or other anti-arthritic drugs, cirrhosis of the liver or sometimes it is the first sign of a carcinoma of the stomach. The amount of blood lost daily is not enough to be detectable as a change in colour in the stools, but over the months it adds up to a significant amount. Sometimes patients have adequate iron reserves in the body but are unable to use them because the marrow is affected by some deep-seated disease like renal failure or rheumatoid arthritis, in which case giving iron does not help much.

If the marrow is starved of iron it responds by putting less haemoglobin into each erythrocyte, so the cells become slightly pale (*hypochromic*). It also makes each cell slightly smaller than usual, these being termed *microcytes*, and these two features are diagnostic of iron deficiency anaemia when seen under a microscope.

The early features of iron deficiency are quite subtle and include weariness and fatigue, anorexia and poor resistance to infection. In children the desire for strange substances such as coal or chalk may be the first sign, known as *pica* (L = magpie). Later, the mucus membranes look pale, the tongue becomes smooth and sore with *glossitis* and the nails crack and become brittle and *spoon-shaped*. Finally there is breathlessness, insomnia, palpitations, angina and difficulty swallowing in some, although many of these symptoms are common and not necessarily due to anaemia. In time of doubt an estimate of the haemoglobin content of the blood and the discovery of hypochromic microcytes will confirm the diagnosis.

PERNICIOUS ANAEMIA

For many years it had been known that in middle age some people quite suddenly began to develop *indigestion* and *glossitis* with a sore tongue and cracked lips, and then a year or so later became very pale and slightly *jaundiced*, finally succumbing to a form of *paralysis*. So resistant was the condition to treatment of any kind that it was known as 'pernicious anaemia', and it was Addison who first observed the connection between the stomach and the anaemia, and whose name is still attached to the disease. However, it was not until 1954 that the role of *intrinsic factor* from the peptic cells of the stomach was established as the missing link in the chain. For it is intrinsic factor which binds the B12 to itself and facilitates absorption in the small intestine, and without it this vitamin simply passes on through.

Pernicious anaemia is very seldom due to dietary deficiency, as the body only requires minute amounts of vitamin B12 and has a large store of it in the liver which lasts several years. In some people, however, the peptic cells of the stomach atrophy around the age of 40–60, and cease to produce both intrinsic factor and acid, so the early symptoms are those of dyspepsia due to achlorhydria. This atrophy is often familial and is usually due to an autoimmune process, so antibodies to the gastric cells are found in the blood. The individuals are typically fair and blue-eyed but with a lemon tinge to the skin on account of the mild jaundice.

Vitamin B12 contains the element cobalt and is essential for the construction of the wall of the erythrocyte in the marrow, as well as maintaining the well-being of the myelin sheath of the nerves of the spinal cord. If this vitamin is not available the cell wall is thin and fragile and breaks down prematurely after about a quarter of its life span. This releases excess bilirubin into the blood and causes a constant slight jaundice. The cells also end up a size too large and are termed *macrocytes* or, when immature, *megaloblasts*, in contrast to the microcytes of iron deficiency. If diagnosis of the condition is delayed, the spinal cord will start to *demyelinate* causing tingling, weakness and loss of reflexes in the feet and legs, followed eventually by similar damage to the brain in the form of *dementia*. Because the problem is essentially one of deficiency it is eminently treatable by giving B12 by injection (to by-pass the absent intrinsic factor), but any neurological damage already sustained unfortunately cannot be repaired.

Folic acid, so called because it was first obtained from foliage, is another B vitamin required for the construction of mature erythrocytes. It is present in adequate amounts in most diets, but *pregnancy* makes heavy demands on the body's reserves and supplements may be needed. If they are not forthcoming then the marrow makes the larger megaloblasts and these work less efficiently, but deficiency of this vitamin does not lead to the neurological consequences of B12 deficiency.

HAEMOLYTIC ANAEMIAS – SICKLE CELL AND THALASSAEMIA

Not all anaemia is due to a deficiency in production of cells, some types of anaemia are caused by premature breakdown of the erythrocyte before its allotted time span (about 120 days), a process called *haemolysis*. This leads to the liberation of large amounts of iron which is retained for further use, as well as the formation of quantities of bilirubin which is carried to the liver for use in the bile and leads to a degree of jaundice in the body (the megaloblastic anaemias are also examples of this as we have seen). The increase in turnover only becomes a problem if the breakdown of cells exceeds the regenerative capacity of the marrow when a *haemolytic crisis* occurs against a background of haemolytic anaemia.

Most haemolytic anaemias are inherited defects of red cell stability, either because the envelope of the cell is the wrong shape (*spherocytosis*) or because the haemoglobin within is abnormal in some way (*haemoglobinopathy*). It is the latter which is responsible for the two conditions of *thalassaemia* and *sickle cell anaemia.*

Normal haemoglobin consists of a four-armed structure, each arm containing an atom of iron and a chain of about 150 amino acids coiled around it. The four arms are arranged in two pairs with two identical alpha chains on one side and two beta chains on the other. The exact nature and sequence of the amino acids in the chain is determined genetically and of critical importance to the successful functioning of the molecule, so when they are incorrect the result is that less oxygen can be carried and the cell wall may also collapse.

Sickle cell anaemia is one such inherited condition found mainly among those of black African descent. It is likely that the disease has persisted throughout generations because of the significant protection the abnormal haemoglobin gives against malaria. One or both of the side chains of the molecule contains substituted amino acids and this leads to the *trait* or the *disease* respectively. In the case of sickle cell trait there is little evidence of anaemia, and it is only the presence of two abnormal side chains which leads to real problems in the form of sickle cell disease, inherited from two parents with the trait. Here the anaemia is severe and comes on a few months after birth, when many of the children die. Those who survive develop an *enlarged liver and spleen* to cope with the increasing turnover and their lives are punctuated with severe *bone pains* when a haemolytic crisis occurs and the tissue is deprived of blood and dies.

Thalassaemia inherits its name from the occurrence in races which inhabit the Mediterranean shores (Gr. thalassa = sea), although it is also widespread in parts of Asia. There is reluctance on the part of the marrow to synthesize adequate amounts of adult haemoglobin, so that which is used is mostly of the foetal type and therefore rapidly destroyed. Foetal haemoglobin is of a slightly different specification for use in the uterus and is normally discarded soon after birth and adult haemoglobin substituted (hence the incidence of a degree of jaundice in most babies at the time of birth).

Where it persists to only a slight degree the condition of *thalassaemia minor* is said to occur and, like the sickle cell trait, there is little actual disability. *Thalassaemia major* entails severe anaemia with the marrow enlarging as it struggles to maintain supplies, causing prominence of the bones of the skull and face as well as hypertrophy of the liver and spleen to dispose of the breakdown products (indeed the spleen is often surgically removed in an attempt to slow down the process of destruction).

POLYCYTHAEMIA

This condition of too many red cells in the circulation is found under normal physiological conditions in those living at high altitude when the low oxygen content of the air stimulates the marrow. An analogous situation may happen in the event of *chronic respiratory disease* when there is less oxygen in the blood and a similar stimulus is evoked. This is because the kidney cells are underoxygenated and respond by secreting larger amounts of the hormone *erythropoietin* which stimulates the bone marrow.

However, in the condition of *primary polycythaemia*, sometimes called 'polycythaemia rubra vera', there is an apparently unprovoked increase in the quantity of erythrocytes in the blood which may reach large numbers and cause an increase in the viscosity, slowing down the circulation and encouraging the blood to clot in the veins. Earlier symptoms are headaches and dizziness, itching of the skin and a flushed face. The blood pressure is elevated and the congestion leads sometimes to bleeding or menorrhagia, so that it may be necessary to remove a pint of blood from the circulation every few weeks. The cause of the disease is not known, but some cases go on to develop a form of leukaemia after many years.

WHITE CELL DISORDERS

The white cells circulating in the blood are mainly *granulocytes* (also called *myelocytes* from the Greek word myelos meaning marrow), *lymphocytes* and a few *monocytes*. However, there are many other white cells in the lymphatic system in the form of *lymphocytes*, and disorders of these stationary white cells, such as *lymphoma* and *myeloma* were discussed in Chapter 2. Unlike erythrocytes, the leucocytes are only very rarely depleted in a condition called *agranulocytosis*, when the marrow stops producing them because of suppression by drugs or infection. More commonly, though still only affecting about 1 person in 10,000, the marrow overproduces either lymphocytes or myelocytes (granulocytes) and results in leukaemia.

LEUKAEMIA

The number of white cells produced by the marrow varies widely and may suddenly increase in the presence of infection, so the marrow may be

95

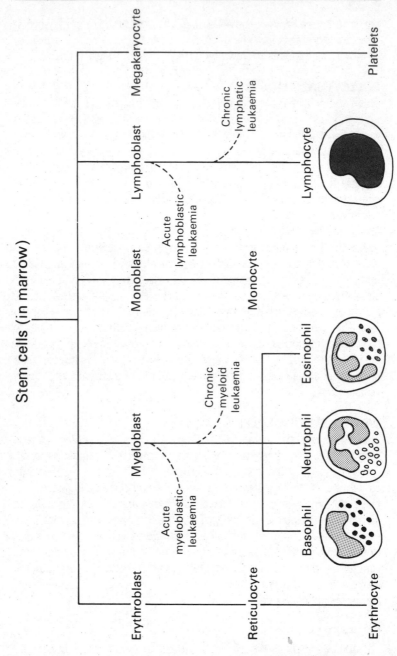

FIGURE 8.1   *Development of blood cells showing the origin of leukaemias*

called upon to work overtime. All the different types of cells in the blood derive ultimately from a single type of cell in the marrow called the *stem cell* by a process of differentiation followed by maturation, and during the maturation process the early cells are termed 'blast' forms (Gr. blastos = bud), as illustrated in figure 8.2. Leukaemia is a form of cancer caused by the uncontrolled multiplication of a single one of these white cells at some stage in its process of maturation, and the symptoms of the disease picture therefore differ according to how mature or primitive that leucocyte was when it began to get out of control.

Thus *acute lymphatic leukaemia* is a form of leukaemia affecting the lymphatic cells at an early stage of maturation when they are still lymphoblasts, and the leukaemic cell is quite primitive and undifferentiated and therefore more destructive. This means that it is a sudden, acute condition and is seen in young children in whom huge numbers of ineffectual lymphoblasts in the marrow crowd out the production of erythrocytes and thrombocytes as well as the other white cell series. This leads to the symptoms of *anaemia* and *pallor, bruising* and *bleeding gums*. There will also be a series of *recurrent infections* such as sore throats and pneumonia. The lymphocytes occupy not only the blood but also the lymph nodes, causing them to swell, as well as enlarging the liver and spleen.

Acute myeloid leukaemia involves people of a much older age group, usually those over 60, and is a rarer disease. Many of the symptoms are similar to those of acute lymphoblastic leukaemia, but there is less swelling of the lymphatic tissue. Because no effective neutrophils are available *infections* set in early and can be rampant, sometimes overwhelming the patient before the diagnosis is made.

Chronic lymphatic and *chronic myeloid leukaemia* are altogether slower processes whereby the cells produced, though malignant, are very much more mature and thus go some way to serving the needs of the body. It may be a matter of years rather than weeks before the symptoms become apparent and the condition diagnosed, and they happen very gradually. The sufferer is usually an elderly person and the anaemia, lymphatic enlargement and general ill-health pass unnoticed for a while. They may develop night sweats and weight loss, culminating in an infection, and the disease smoulders on for many years before finally gathering pace and changing to the acute type of leukaemia.

CLOTTING DISORDERS
Blood clotting is a complex process involving a number of chemical and cellular chain reactions before the clot is finally formed. In many patients

coagulation may occur too readily and lead to a thrombosis in a vital vessel and such people are often treated with *anticoagulant drugs* such as Warfarin to slow this process down. Because it is vital that some clotting ability is retained periodic checks of their 'clotting time' must be made and the dose adjusted if necessary.

It is possible on rare occasions for one of these clotting factors to be absent, and this defect is inherited. One such is *haemophilia* which, though rare, is perhaps the best known. This particular disorder affects only men, being inherited on the sex chromosome, and in those who have it there can be extensive bleeding after a cut and large *ecchymoses* after minor trauma. Sometimes bleeding occurs internally, especially into the joints which may become damaged and arthritic in adulthood. The missing *factor VIII* is given by regular injection on a prophylactic basis, with additional doses administered when necessary if an accident occurs which requires further treatment. Because factor VIII is concentrated from pooled human plasma which is then removed as a 'cryoprecipitate', that is a fraction which condenses at a certain temperature, prior to 1985 there was a high risk of contamination with HI virus, and many haemophiliacs contracted AIDS this way. Blood products are now heat treated to eliminate this risk.

Thrombocytopenia, or lack of sufficient thrombocytes in the blood, leads eventually to a similar situation of bleeding after trauma, but usually there is earlier evidence that the number of thrombocytes in the blood are gradually falling. This takes the form of widespread tiny bruises known as *petechiae* in the skin. The falling count is due to widespread self-destruction of blood platelets by an auto-immune process, and this may happen either spontaneously – *idiopathic thrombocytopenic purpura* – or as a side effect of certain drugs.

CHAPTER NINE

HEART:
DISORDERS OF
PROPULSION

*T*he heart is more than a pump, it is also the seat of the emotions and the location in the body where we identify our feelings. We speak of someone as warm-hearted or stony-hearted, in grief our hearts break and in fear or excitement they miss a beat. Because of this intimate awareness of the heart there is often a concern about heart disease and this may create actual symptoms in some people, especially those who have been recently bereaved. These symptoms usually take the form of a nagging discomfort in the left side of the chest, palpitations and sometimes some difficulty breathing. They can be very similar to those caused by the major cause of death in the UK, *coronary heart disease*, so the fears are sometimes justifiable and the two must be carefully distinguished.

Since the turn of the century there has been a steady increase in the number of heart attacks in the developed world, and heart disease now accounts for one third of all deaths in the UK for reasons which are discussed below. There is an exact correlation between the level of cholesterol in the blood and the death rate in any given country, and in this we are near the top of the international league table, exceeded only by the Finns and the Irish. In the US and Australia the incidence of heart attacks has halved since 1970 as dietary customs have altered, and recently the statistics in the UK have also begun to improve a little.

THE PATHOLOGY OF CORONARY HEART DISEASE
By the early teens most of us have already developed the very first evidence of narrowing of the arteries which starts as deposits of white, fatty streaks of cholesterol on the intimal layer of the major arteries. Over the years, at a rate largely in accordance with the factors listed in table 9.1, these streaks mature into thickened *plaques* which project into the lumen of the vessel and narrow it, reducing the circulation to a trickle. Eventually the plaques may ulcerate and the turbulence in the blood flow allows the build up of clumps of platelets which eventually block the vessel. This process is not just happening in the coronary arteries, but any diminution of the blood flow here is likely to

have the most dramatic consequences. The immediate result is *ischaemia*, or lack of blood flow to the organ supplied, in this case the *myocardium*. If the ischaemia builds up slowly over the years then the result is a gradual loss of efficiency in the organ until it fails to operate, but if the blood flow terminates abruptly then the results can be catastrophic, as happens in a heart attack.

The early pathologists, who were a down-to-earth lot, called these deposits of cholesterol 'porridge', but they were also versed in the classics so they used the Greek term *atheroma*, and later *atherosclerosis* (which means 'hard porridge'). It is atherosclerosis which is responsible for a plethora of pathology in the form of strokes, gangrene of the feet and renal failure as well as myocardial ischaemia, depending on which vessels are most involved.

The average British diet is composed of about 40% fat (lipid), of which 95% is in the form of *triglycerides*. Chemically triglycerides are made up of a central core of glycerol to which three fatty acids are attached, and these fatty acids can be either saturated, monounsaturated or polyunsaturated, depending on the type of food. In general animal fats tend to be more of the saturated variety, and it is these which lead

TABLE 9.1	Risk factors in ischaemic heart disease
Cholesterol Level	Extremely significant, diet related
Triglyceride Level	Significant, diet related
Smoking	Directly depends on number & duration
Blood Pressure	Increases dramatically if diastolic >110
Family History	Very significant
Obesity	Significant
Stress	Increased risk in the driving, ambitious person
Exercise	Increases chance of survival by improving circuln.
Fish Intake	Contains linoleic acid which protects
Fibre Intake	Protects
Coffee Intake	More than 5 cups/day may increase risk slightly
Alcohol Intake	Small quantity protects, large quantity exposes
Oral Contraceptives	Increases risk slightly
Diabetes	Increases risk of atherosclerosis generally
Myxoedema	Increases risk of atherosclerosis generally

especially to atheroma. Olive oil is a good source of monounsaturated fat, while sunflower and safflower oils contain the highest quantity of polyunsaturates.

Of even greater significance, however, is the level of circulating *cholesterol* in the plasma, for this is a necessary component of cell membranes, bile salts and steroid hormones. As well as being synthesised by the liver it is present in meat, eggs and dairy products, so a diet rich in these can result in excessive levels in the body. Cholesterol and triglycerides are transported in the blood attached to proteins known as the lipoproteins and these differ in density, the lower density lipoproteins (LDL) carrying the cholesterol and the high density lipoproteins (HDL) the triglycerides. In assessing the risk of excessive fat, or hyperlipidaemia, to the individual, what is measured is both the cholesterol and the lipoproteins, and in particular the ratio of the HDL to the LDL. A few unfortunates inherit a very high level of lipoproteins which renders them extremely susceptible to heart disease, but for the majority of us it is a case of changing our eating habits.

ANGINA PECTORIS

If the supply of blood (and hence oxygen) to the heart muscle should decline, a cramp-like pain in the chest develops, known as *angina*. This is felt at times of physical and emotional stress when the heart's demand for blood is highest, but anaemia may sometimes bring it on. The amount of exertion needed is similar with each attack, so the patient soon learns to anticipate when to ease up. Walking against a cold wind is especially provocative but heavy meals or smoking can also precipitate angina. One useful diagnostic sign is that angina comes on during, not after exercise, and is relieved by rest within a few minutes.

The *character* of the pain is typical and is felt as a dull, tight, constricting pain, occasionally an ache but never a sharp, stabbing pain. It may easily be mistaken for indigestion as the ache may be in the lower chest and even be accompanied by belching. The *distribution* of the pain varies, but is always the same in an individual and usually starts behind the sternum (*retrosternal pain*) but cannot accurately be located by pointing. It may radiate down the inside of the left or even occasionally the right arm to the hand, ending in the 4th and 5th fingers. In a few it may be felt in the jaw, the back or the upper abdomen.

A particularly serious type of angina is that known as *unstable angina*, as this may herald the onset of a *heart attack*. It is recognised by an increase in the severity of the pain and a change in its radiation pattern. The pain may come on spontaneously and fluctuate for several days and then end or go on to become an attack, and it is patients who develop these symptoms who are usually offered surgery in the form of a bypass graft, using a vein removed from the leg in the hope that this will prevent an infarction (see below).

HEART ATTACK

Many of those with angina can continue a relatively normal life, limited only at the extremes of exercise. A few, however, will at some stage develop a complete occlusion of a coronary vessel by a clot of blood (*thrombosis*) which forms on a disrupted plaque of atheroma. Any roughness or ulceration of an artery tends to attract platelets which form a 'seal' over the area, and this in turn leads to superimposed thrombosis and spasm. This denies the muscle cells beyond any source of nourishment, and within 1–2 hours they swell and die. The rate at which this happens depends on the degree of activity of the sympathetic nervous system and the presence of collateral vessels (which previous exercise will tend to enhance greatly). The dead tissue becomes filled with coagulated blood which turns dark red and comes to resemble a piece of salami, so has been

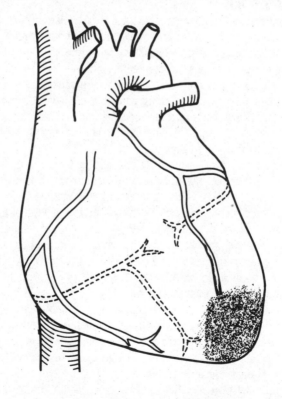

FIGURE 9.1   *Myocardial infarction*

endowed with the delightful name of *infarction* (from the Latin infarcere = stuffing). This *myocardial infarction*, to give it the correct name, will then proceed to contract and eventually become a scar (assuming that the patient survives the assault) but until it has done so the heart and circulation are at some risk of certain complications which may ensue.

The attacks usually arrive without warning, often during sleep, and cause a severe pain which is similar in distribution to angina but much more severe, sometimes causing *sweating, nausea, vomiting* and *extreme fear*. The pain comes on over a period of several minutes and lasts much longer than angina and may go on for several hours without stopping. In one third of cases the attack follows unstable angina, and some develop an infarction at the height of some strenuous activity. In about one in ten (usually the elderly) a 'silent coronary' occurs, when there is no pain at all but only sweating, dizziness and breathlessness. In general, the greater the amount of myocardial damage the more severe are the symptoms.

The complications depend to a large extent on which coronary artery was involved and hence where the infarct occurred. Another factor is whether the full thickness of the myocardium was damaged or just the endocardial or pericardial layers. Obviously in the case of a massive infarction which follows a major blockage the chances of death are high, and this is the outcome in about 40% of cases, one third of whom will perish immediately.

If the person survives, however, the pumping power of the heart will usually be impaired to some degree, and be too feeble to maintain enough pressure to supply the tissues which therefore become cold, pale and clammy. The patient is said to be in *cardiogenic shock* with a low blood pressure and rapid feeble pulse. The injured left ventricle may have difficulty expelling all the blood it receives, and some will get held up in the lungs causing *pulmonary oedema* and breathlessness, one of the early signs of *heart failure* (see below).

Even if the patient does not succumb to the immediate attack they are still not out of the wood, and another third die within the first 48 hours. The usual reason for this is the involvement of the conduction pathways of the heart which are damaged in the infarction, so that an *arrythmia* or irregular rhythm occurs and the heart starts to beat in a wild or erratic fashion. These arrythmias are broadly speaking of two kinds, those involving the atria only and those involving the ventricles, and it is for this reason that patients are monitored with a cardiograph continuously in hospital. If the disruption is near the beginning of the conducting system, in the atria, then these will either beat very fast (*atrial flutter*) or irregularly (*atrial fibrillation*). The pulse will accordingly be rapid but regular at about 150/minute in the case of flutter, or totally irregular if there is atrial fibrillation.

However, these atrial abnormalities are much less ominous than arrhythmias which arise in the ventricles. Here the impulse may be entirely blocked in its passage, so the heart beats very slowly at the rate set by the ventricles of about 40–50 a minute, known as *heart block*, and it is in situations like this that a temporary packemaker may be required. Or new *ectopic beats* arise from a spontaneous source and these may become so rapid that they lead to *ventricular fibrillation* with the ventricles just quivering but unable to pump. Defibrillation can be attempted by applying an electric shock to the heart which temporarily stuns it and then usually allows normal rhythm to return.

As the wall of the ventricle heals a few weeks later, it may on occasions bulge outwards to form a swelling known as an *aneurysm* (Gr = dilation), and this will obviously impair the efficiency with which the heart pumps, leading to heart failure. If the infarction involves the inner lining of the heart, the endocardium, then this becomes roughened and attracts a clot of blood to stick to it, a *mural thrombus*, which may later break off and enter the circulation as an *embolus* (Gr = wedge). These emboli can end up anywhere in the systemic circulation, perhaps in the brain or leg to interfere with the blood supply there and possibly cause an infarction of those tissues. Finally the outer layer or pericardium may be involved in the infarction and become inflamed, leading to *pericarditis*. If this happens there is a recurrence of the pain a few days later, but this time a sharper, stabbing pain accompanied by a slight fever (the post-myocardial infarction syndrome).

BLOOD PRESSURE

The heart pumps blood around the body under pressure which varies according to the phase of the cardiac cycle, and this is felt at the wrist as a pulse wave. The highest pressure in the vessel coincides with the systolic phase of the ventricle and so is called the *systolic pressure*, and gives a measure of the force with which the heart is beating at the time and varies according to the needs of the body. The trough of the pulse wave occurs when the heart relaxes and is therefore termed the *diastolic pressure*. Even during diastole a flow is maintained in the arteries because of the elastic quality of their walls, so the diastolic pressure is the more significant of the two measurements and reflects the state of the arterioles and their ability to relax.

Several factors influence our BP. The immediate one is the

contractile force of the heart. so if the blood supply to the myocardium is defective it may be unable to contract forcefully and the BP drops suddenly to cause shock as we have already seen. Secondly the *volume of blood* which has to be pumped will influence the pressure, which also drops if we suddenly start to haemorrhage, but equally increases if our blood volume should increase for any reason. The usual reason is that our body contains an excessive amount of salt, since our kidneys have evolved to conserve this valuable mineral and are reluctant to part with it. An average diet contains far more salt than is necessary, and in order to dilute it water is retained by the body and increases the volume of plasma which in turn elevates the blood pressure. The Chinese Yellow Emperor, Huang Ti, referred to this when he noted that people who ate salt had hard pulses.

Thirdly the *peripheral resistance* of the arterioles can modify the BP considerably. This is done by constricting or dilating the muscular walls by a change in autonomic tone under the control of the vasomotor centre in the brain, which is in turn influenced by emotional factors such as anxiety, stress etc. All these factors serve to adjust our BP to the varying needs of the body at different times, but sometimes the mechanism malfunctions and *hypertension* ensues and slowly damages certain organs.

Causes of Hypertension

About 90% of those with high blood pressure have *primary essential hypertension* which means that they have no demonstrable abnormality in any bodily system and the direct cause of their condition is a combination of the factors mentioned above. Some will have a family history of 'blood pressure', some will be overweight but many are outwardly fit and healthy with no signs of anything amiss. It is often assumed that headaches are caused by blood pressure, but in fact this is seldom the case except in the rare instance of malignant hypertension (see below), and very often damage is caused without the person being aware.

If the kidneys become diseased they respond by secreting increased amounts of the hormone *renin*, whose function is to constrict the arterial walls and so elevate the pressure in the vessels. Many kidney diseases thus engender a degree of hypertension, particularly *nephritis, chronic pyelitis, polycystic kidneys* and probably to a degree in *toxaemia of pregnancy*. Certain hormonal abnormalities, such as an excess of cortisone in *Cushing's syndrome*, or of thyroxine in thyrotoxicosis or of oestrogens in the case of oral contraceptives in some who are susceptible will also bring about what is known as *secondary hypertension* but this is not, however, the usual cause of high blood pressure.

Consequences of Hypertension

Until the condition has been present for a good number of years and one of the target organs like the heart, brain or kidney is affected there are no symptoms apparent and the condition cannot be diagnosed unless someone takes the blood pressure (see below). Eventually the *left ventricle* of the heart enlarges or *hypertrophies* to produce the extra power required and this may be detectable clinically as a heaving impulse on the left border of the chest. By then the blood supply to the myocardium is often inadequate and the heart begins to fail, the patient experiencing breathlessness from the accumulating pulmonary oedema, and sometimes even sustaining a *myocardial infarction*. The other main organ affected is the brain, in which the increased pressure may lead to a *stroke* (see chapter 17) especially in the elderly in whom the vessels are somewhat hard and brittle.

A more sinister type of hypertension sometimes arises in younger people when the blood pressure rapidly accelerates to very high levels in the space of a few weeks and causes severe headaches and visual problems. This is known as *malignant hypertension* and is usually fatal within a few months unless promptly treated. Because the patient is young the heart is able to withstand the greatly elevated pressure, and the brunt of the attack falls on the kidneys which become congested and go into *renal failure*. There is a marked thickening in the inner layer of the larger renal arterioles which therefore fail to supply the glomeruli and these atrophy, a change which is mirrored in the retina and can be directly observed with the opthalmoscope.

Taking Blood Pressure

This is done by wrapping a cuff around the upper arm and occluding the artery using an instrument called a *sphygmomanometer* (Gr. sphingo = throttle, the Sphinx was a monster who throttled her victims). The pressure is then lowered until a soft, tapping sound is just heard, caused by the turbulence of the blood in the narrowed artery, and this signifies the systolic pressure. As the cuff continues to deflate the distortion of the artery lessens and the turbulence becomes a smooth flow so that eventually the sound disappears altogether, at the point where the normal contours of the artery have been regained. This represents the diastolic pressure and is sometimes heard as a muffling of the sound rather than its disappearance.

If problems arise it is probably because a) the stethoscope has not been placed exactly over the brachial artery (or even has the hole occluded), b) the elbow is bent or has a tight sleeve over it, c) the arm is very fat which makes accuracy difficult, d) the valve in the sphygmomano-meter has not been unscrewed/screwed up or e) you have not had enough practice! If a high reading is obtained then it should be checked when the practitioner and the patient have rested quietly for a few minutes.

Interpreting Blood Pressure

In Western societies, both the systolic and the diastolic pressure tends to increase gradually with age, whereas in communities where the consumption of salt is minimal there appears to be no fluctuation of pressure during life. The maximal accepted values for the systolic pressure are generally regarded as the age of the patient plus 100, measured in mm of mercury, so the systolic pressure of a young person would be up to about 130 mm, although it must be remembered that this will vary widely according to circumstances. As regards the diastolic pressure there is less agreement about the level at which the label 'abnormal' should be applied, but the graph in figure 9.2 gives an indication of average readings and it is well to be suspicious of levels of over 100.

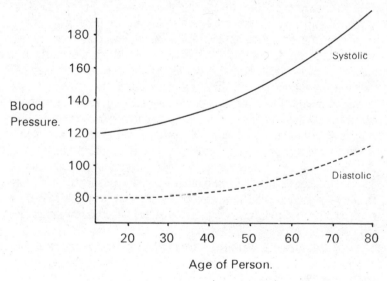

FIGURE 9.2   *Upper limit of systolic and diastolic pressures*

HEART FAILURE

When the heart is unable to perform its primary function of pumping blood to the tissues it is said to have failed, but as the pump is a double one things are not quite so straightforward since the left ventricle ejects at a pressure of about 120 mm of Hg, whereas the right is only operating at a pressure of about 25 mm. Moreover, as we have seen, the left ventricle is much more frequently affected by ischaemic heart disease and hypertension, so it is this one which usually fails – *left ventricular failure* or *LVF*. Failure of a chamber of the heart has two consequences, firstly insufficient pressure is generated to perfuse the tissues ahead, sometimes called 'forward failure', but also excessive quantities of blood are held back and clog up the tissues behind (backward failure). So we can see that there are two groups of symptoms involved with each type of failure.

Left Ventricular Failure is usually the result of *ischaemia* or *hypertension*, less commonly *valvular disease* or *cardiomyopathy*. It is also the natural consequence of old age in a heart which beats about 28 billion times in the average lifetime, so breathlessness (dyspnoea) on exertion comes to us all in time. This is because blood which cannot be pumped through the left ventricle queues up in the lungs and congests the lung capillaries, preventing the rapid diffusion of oxygen. The high pressure in the capillaries causes plasma to leak into the alveoli and the lungs become congested and provoke the slight cough so common in the elderly.

While the person is up and about during the day, most of this congestion occurs at the base of the lungs and is not too much of a problem, apart from some breathlessness (*dyspnoea*) on exertion. However, after a few hours in bed, the slowing of the heart coupled with the redistribution of the fluid throughout the lung fields may cause him or her to wake gasping for breath with severe dyspnoea and a wet cough with pink, frothy sputum. This is known as *acute LVF* or *cardiac asthma* on account of the wheeze, which is caused by the airways filling with oedema fluid. Some relief is obtained by sitting upright (orthopnoea) so that the fluid drains back to the base of the lungs, and they usually prefer to sit by an open window. In sudden, severe cardiac asthma, such as is caused by an acute myocardial infarction, there is pallor, faintness, sweating and cyanosis.

Right Ventricular Failure. Sooner or later the congested capillaries of the lungs resulting from left ventricular failure will exert a back pressure on the right ventricle, and failure of the right side of the heart will follow. Or it sometimes happens that the right ventricle alone is affected by ischaemia or valvular disease and is unable to pump blood into the lungs. In this case the back pressure will be exerted on blood in the peripheral veins, particularly those in the feet, and so the first sign is usually oedema of the ankles which start to swell (although swollen ankles also arise from other causes such as varicose veins). Over a long period organs nearer to the heart become involved, especially those such as the liver which possess an extensive network of capillaries, and these likewise become congested to cause enlargement of the organ and even, eventually, cirrhosis. The back pressure also travels into the jugular veins in the neck which become visibly distended with a pulse that rises and falls with the heartbeat.

Many cases of right sided heart failure are not due to pathology in the heart at all, but occur because the circulation of blood through the lungs is impeded by lung diseases, especially chronic bronchitis and emphysema (see chapter 11), or sometimes a pulmonary embolus (see chapter 10). The pressure in the pulmonary circulation then rises in a manner similar to that which occurs in the systemic circulation in essential hypertension, and is therefore termed *pulmonary hypertension*. This will cause the right ventricle to enlarge until it can no longer cope and begins to fail. To this state of affairs the rather quaint phrase *cor pulmonale* has been given, meaning literally 'heart from the lungs', in other words heart disease secondary to lung disease.

Congestive Heart Failure. Although pure right or left sided heart failure does occur, it must be remembered that as both sides work together it is common for a degree of each to coexist and the term congestive heart failure is then used. The reason for this is that several conditions, such as anaemia and thyrotoxicosis, cause an increased demand for blood from both sides equally, so they fail together. Secondly, because the kidney responds to a lack of blood perfusion by retaining salt and water, this compounds the problem and causes a general increase in fluid retention by the body. It is for this reason that dietary salt restriction is desirable, and why diuretics are usually used in orthodox treatment.

PERICARDITIS

This is an inflammatory condition of the pericardium, due to *infection, neoplasm, myocardial infarction* or sometimes *rheumatoid arthritis*. The usual cause is a virus, when it may follow a chest infection especially in young men. The pain is accompanied by a fever, and is felt as a sharp pain over the front of the chest, sometimes referred to the left shoulder as well. It is made worse by deep inspiration and lying down on the left side. If the inflammation is severe, the roughened surfaces can be heard with a stethoscope, like a tree creaking in the wind in time with the heartbeat – the *friction rub*. Pericarditis not uncommonly follows a few days after a myocardial infarction, and may also be a feature of a bronchial carcinoma which is extending directly towards the heart.

In certain cases, especially cancer of the bronchus, a collection of fluid called a *pericardial effusion* may accumulate quite rapidly within the pericardium and compress the heart so that it cannot pump adequately and begins to fail. If this is caused by a tubercular infection, a very rigid and thickened pericardium may result, called *constrictive pericarditis*, and produce similar symptoms.

RHEUMATIC FEVER

Fifty years ago the phrase 'acute rheumatism' was regarded as an ominous portent of heart disease to come and synonymous with what is now more often termed *rheumatic fever*. It is a condition which tends to affect children and adolescents, and although much less common now it is still a scourge of the developing world and responsible for most heart disease there. The decrease in this country started well before the advent of antibiotics and probably reflects changes in the virulence of the *haemolytic streptococcus*, the organism which is intimately related to the condition. For the fever is preceded 2–3 weeks before by an infection of the bacterium, usually in the throat, and this stimulates the production of antibodies by the lymph glands. Unfortunately these antibodies then go on to attack the connective tissues of the heart and joints, which by

TABLE 9.1 Possible causes of chest pain

Condition	Pointers
Angina pectoris	Character, during effort, radiation, temporary
Myocardial infarction	Character, often at rest, sweating, vomiting
Cardiac neurosis	Left inframammary, aching, after effort, tense
Tracheitis	Cough, scratchy pain, localised
Pleurisy	Local, peripheral, sharp, worse on inspiration
Hiatus hernia	Burning pain, reflux, after meals, worse lying
Pulmonary embolus	Sharp pain, fainting, haemoptysis, dyspnoea
Herpes zoster	Single dermatome, rash later
Bronchial carcinoma	Smoker, cough, weight loss, sharp pain
Bornholm disease	Fever, headache, lower chest aches, tender muscles
Aortic aneurysm	Sudden, tearing, shock, abdominal swelling
Pneumothorax	Abrupt onset, sharp stab, breathlessness
Osteoarthritis	Age, posture, recurrence in certain position
Osteoporosis	Age, kyphosis, worse on movement, girdle pain
Pericarditis	Sharp pain, fever, worse movement & inspiration
Referred pain	Peptic ulcer, cholecystitis, hepatitis, splenomegaly

coincidence have a protein structure identical to that of part of the streptococcus.

The first symptoms of rheumatic fever are an abrupt *arthritis* which flits from one large joint to another every few days, accompanied by sweating and a rapid pulse. At the same time the heart is also being damaged in the process, leading to heart failure and breathlessness when the myocardium is involved, but also attacking the valves to give rise to small growths and irregularities on them. These interfere with the flow of blood through the heart and cause turbulence which is heard as a *heart murmur* and over the months, as the acute inflammation dies down, the valve becomes permanently deformed and fibrotic – *rheumatic heart disease*. The valve most frequently affected is the mitral valve, and also to a lesser extent the aortic, and these may either end up narrowed – *stenosis*, or leaking and unable to close properly – *incompetent*. The long-term consequences of this are that back pressure will congest the lungs and eventually even the right ventricle, so various operations have been devised for restructuring or replacing the affected valves.

The acute disease, which as the saying goes 'licks the joints but bites the heart', is not confined to these two organs alone, and lesions appear sometimes on the skin as the typical rash of *erythema marginatum*. This is an erythema, or reddening of the skin, in patches which have a distinct margin, so that they look a little like ringworm without the scaling. A more frequent feature are the *subcutaneous nodules* seen on the bony protuberances such as the elbows and knees. These are painless swellings under the skin such as are also seen in rheumatoid arthritis. Another distinctive feature sometimes seen is *Sydenham's chorea* (not to be confused with Huntington's chorea, an inherited disability). The word comes from the Greek 'chorus', which was the dance performed during a play, and describes the spontaneous writhing and twisting movements which take place for a few days. In their mild state they may not amount to much and be mistaken for fidgetting and restlessness, so many cases of rheumatic fever are only diagnosed retrospectively when the heart murmur is noticed or the patient becomes breathless.

CONGENITAL HEART DISEASE

Not all heart murmurs are rheumatic in origin, however, and about 1 in 100 babies are born with a persistent heart murmur of whom a quarter have a defect serious enough to require surgery. The heart develops from a series of folds in the main blood vessel during the seventh week of embryonic life and minor irregularities easily occur, usually for no apparent reason but sometimes as a result of maternal infections such as rubella. The common abnormalities are either obstructions to the flow of blood or abnormal communications between the chambers – a 'hole in the heart'.

These latter defects are the most common variety and consist of defects in the septum between the left and right sides of the heart so are called ventricular septal defects (VSD) or atrial septal defects (ASD) accordingly. They range from minute pinhole-size apertures to holes large enough to *'shunt'* much of the blood across from the left to the right ventricle each time the heart beats, flooding the lungs with blood and causing cyanosis (the 'blue baby'). As the child gets older most of these holes tend to diminish in size, but some of the larger ones will need an operation to protect the lungs from future damage from pulmonary hypertension.

Stenosis or narrowing may also occur, principally to the pulmonary valve which may eventually cause the right side of the heart to fail, or to the aortic arch itself, when it is known as *'coarctation of the aorta'*. This is a narrowing of the aorta at any point along its course but usually the arch, and effectively prevents blood reaching the tissues beyond. The heart must therefore generate tremendous pressure in its attempt to push blood through and enlarges to a considerable size unless the obstruction is relieved. For this reason it is important to routinely examine the femoral pulse of all newborn babies as this will be missing in such cases.

CARDIOMYOPATHY

During its lifetime the heart muscle gets through an enormous amount of work, pumping about seven tons of blood every day of our life. It is therefore very susceptible to changes not only in its blood supply but also in its general nutrition. If there is a shortcoming in vitamins, thyroxine or other nutrients, as may occur particularly in alcoholism, the muscle will weaken, the heart dilate, and eventually failure will occur, a state known as *congestive cardiomyopathy*. Another type of cardiomyopathy is congenital in origin and stems from an inability of the cells to contract fully, so they eventually swell up and impede the flow of blood through the heart as *hypertrophic cardiomyopathy*. In both cases there is progressive weakness, dyspnoea and fatigue, with palpitations and irregularities of the heartbeat which may be dangerous.

DRUGS AND THE HEART

The original drug prescribed for heart conditions was digitalis, which was poached from the herbalists who distilled it from foxglove leaves and used it as a cure for dropsy or oedema. It is still widely used and a valuable stimulant, but now synthesized as *lanoxin*. since plant sources varied too widely in their potency, although they did provide many other, often useful, ingredients. Digitalis stimulates the muscles of the heart to beat more forcefully, and so assists the failing myocardium and improves the circulation. It also inhibits the conduction of the impulse through the heart and is thus useful in those with certain irregularities especially atrial fibrillation. However, in slowing the rhythm of the heart it begins to allow spontaneous *ectopic beats* to appear from other sources, mainly the ventricle, and this can be very dangerous and even fatal. Thus the early signs of digitalis overdose are a marked slowing of the heart, followed by coupled beats where an extra ectopic is injected after every normal beat (*pulsus bigeminus*). Because of these risks heart failure is usually treated first with *diuretics* (see chapter 15), and only if these prove inadequate is digitalis used in conjunction with potassium which ensures stability of the heart cells.

Because many of the problems of the heart result from ischaemia or hypertension, it makes more sense to try and relieve these rather than stimulate the heart, and modern heart drugs tend to emphasis this approach. The sympathetic nervous system is responsible for speeding up the rhythm and raising blood pressure by constricting the vessels, so if this can be inhibited many problems are alleviated. Unfortunately the early attempts to block sympathetic tone also blocked its passage to the bronchi, resulting in excessive parasympathetic tone and narrowing of the airways. This was only circumvented by the discovery of two different types of receptor, termed the alpha and beta receptors, the latter applying largely to the cardiovascular system alone. By blocking the beta receptors the blood pressure can be safely lowered and the heart rate slowed, so they are in common use for both angina and hypertension.

There are, however, several provisos to the use of beta blockers. If there is a physical narrowing of the coronary arteries, as happens in ischaemia, the slowing and relaxing of the heart may precipitate a degree of heart failure in those operating at the lower limits of their tolerance, and this may induce some breathlessness. Moreover even the latest 'cardioselective' beta blockers can induce a certain amount of bronchial constriction and should not be used in asthmatics. Nor should beta blockers be withdrawn suddenly, for their cessation can precipitate a rapid worsening of myocardial ischaemia in someone who has been on them for some time.

The side-effects of these drugs are fairly common but generally not dangerous. Patients tend to feel a sleepiness and lack of energy from the reduction in sympathetic tone, and this is sometimes used to 'advantage' in anxiety states and in those who are unable to relax. They may also notice that their hands and feet begin to feel the cold more easily, or a slight dyspepsia. Because certain of the beta blockers are fat soluble they can cross the blood-brain barrier and cause disturbing dreams and nightmares, which go away if the medication is changed.

Hypertension is an area where treatment can be a problem with orthodox medicine, for it is almost inevitably life-long and many of the patients are young at the onset. Other approacches such as salt restriction, weight and especially alcohol reduction, bio-feedback and meditation should be tried as well as complementary approaches. Only if these fail and there is seen to be a real risk should drugs be used. The first used are often diuretics, but they have a relatively mild effect on blood pressure, and usually additional drugs are required.

Beta blockers are themselves used very frequently for hypertension, often with a diuretic in addition. If these are ineffective there are other approaches which can be used, all of them of recent origin. One is to inhibit the movement of calcium within the heart, which is needed to contract the muscle, and this reduces the force of the heart in a manner similar to the beta blockers, but without many of the side effects. These 'calcium antagonists' are exemplified by Verapamil and Nifedipine (Adalat).

Another recent innovation are the ACE inhibitors which reduce blood pressure by inhibiting Angiotensin Converting Enzymes. Angiotensin is the hormone released by the kidney which, as its name suggests, tenses the blood vessels after it has been converted to angiotensin II. They are very effective, very recent and very expensive but are liable to cause such a sudden drop in blood pressure in the initial exposure to the drug that the patient may faint without warning. Should he recover his confidence, however, he will be glad to note that this particular unwanted effect diminishes with the passage of time.

CHAPTER TEN

VESSELS: DISORDERS OF PERFUSION

*E*very part of the body with the exception of the epidermis and the cornea is supplied with blood by a huge network of vessels which stretch for a total of about 75,000 miles in all, enough to go round the world three times! The vast majority of this network is composed of tiny capillaries, but the arteries with their elastic and muscular walls are critical for the regulation of the fluctuating pressure of the heart, yet must not impede the smooth flow of blood. As was indicated in the last chapter, an impediment, if it occurs, is usually in the form of *atheroma*, of which there has been a sevenfold increase since the turn of the century. The onset of atheroma is particularly accelerated in hypertensives and smokers, and also in those who have excess cholesterol in the blood (*hypercholesterolaemia*) either of diabetic, hypothyroid or familial origin.

Atheroma is not the only condition to affect the arteries, however, and as we age deposits of calcium form in the medial coat and lead to 'hardening of the arteries'. To a large extent this is a natural process and does not cause any narrowing of the artery itself but may be felt as thickened, cord-like arteries in elderly people.

THE AORTA

This is the major vessel leaving the heart and as such must bear the brunt of the pressure exerted by the left ventricle. During the last century syphilis was a source of damage to the aorta, and the spirochaete attacked the elastic coat of the artery to weaken it and create an aneurysm in the ascending aorta. This gradually enlarged and compressed the structures of the mediastinum, causing severe deep pains and finally rupturing, sometimes dramatically into the trachea or oesophagus.

Aneurysms of the aorta still occur but of a different type. They affect the descending thoracic or abdominal aorta and cause it either to *bulge* or to *split* so that blood enters the medial coat and 'dissects' it for a short distance before either re-entering the lumen or rupturing through the outer wall leading to rapid death. Such *dissecting*

115

aneurysms occur mainly in middle aged men and cause a severe, tearing pain in the chest and back, accompanied by shock, so they are often misdiagnosed as the more common myocardial infarction.

Another type of abdominal aneurysm, which bulges rather than splits, is due to atheromatous weakening of the whole wall and usually occurs in the abdominal aorta of older people, often without symptoms or with just vague lower back or abdominal pains. A swelling which pulsates will be felt in the abdomen, and this will often remain constant for many years, but will require surgery and a replacement graft if it starts to enlarge. If it occurs in the chest it may press on the trachea or oesophagus and cause a persistent cough or difficulty swallowing.

INTERMITTENT CLAUDICATION

The word 'claudication' means to limp (the Roman emperor Claudius derived his name from this characteristic), and signifies the hallmark of the problem – an aching, cramp-like pain which occurs in the muscles of the calf or foot after walking a short distance, and which is alleviated by resting for a few minutes, only to return on further exertion. This comes about because of the severe narrowing of the femoral or popliteal arteries which may occur in atherosclerosis and is seen usually in men.

The earliest symptoms are cramps in the calves at night, later gradually followed by coldness, blueness and loss of hair over the lower calf. The skin is dry to the touch as sweating is impaired, and when it is blanched by pressure several seconds elapse before the colour is restored. The pulses will often be absent in the foot, knee or groin, depending on the site of the blockage, and eventually the ischaemia becomes so severe that the viability of the skin is affected and it may ulcerate. As the oxygenation of the tissues becomes further compromised, they become blackened and gangrenous and the limb may eventually require amputation. Such a scenario may on rare occasions be seen in young men in their twenties, caused by a reaction to cigarette smoking and termed *Buerger's disease*.

Diabetics are prone to occlusion of particularly the smaller arterioles of the feet, especially if their diabetes is severe and has been badly controlled. Since they are also liable to skin infections, and may have impairment of sensation, the combination not infrequently leads to surgery. So diabetics have to be scrupulous about looking after their feet as the least injury is liable to develop into ulceration.

RAYNAUD'S DISEASE

This is characterised by intermittent episodes of *pallor* and *cyanosis* of the digits, especially the fingers, usually precipitated by exposure to cold or by exercise. The small arteries react by constricting and the fingers turn white, then blue and finally bright red and begin to throb and tingle as the arteries dilate again. It is a genetic condition which is particularly felt by girls and younger women and may sometimes be so severe as to lead to ulceration of the fingertips.

Some patients develop *Raynaud's phenomenon*, which is the same symptom but occurs as a result of some external cause, often a systemic disease of some kind especially collagen diseases such as systemic lupus erythematosis or scleroderma. It may also arise as an unwanted effect of certain drugs such as the beta-blockers given for hypertension or ergot for migraine, or even from the contraceptive pill. Physical damage, too, can lead to Raynaud's phenomenon, such as the use of vibrating machine tools ('white finger') which can cause symptoms for days afterwards. An unusual cause is the presence of an extra rib above the clavicle, a 'cervical rib', which compresses the subclavian artery and can only be diagnosed by taking a chest X-ray.

Chilblains are a more localised form of reaction to the cold and are usually seen on the hands or the feet as areas of swollen and itchy skin which turns red or purple. They may occur in those whose hands get repeatedly chilled and then warmed too quickly in front of a fire.

TEMPORAL ARTERITIS

Although not common, it is very important not to overlook this condition, which is also known as *cranial* or *giant cell arteritis*. It is an inflammatory disorder of the arteries of the head, especially the temporal artery, which can be felt just in front of the ear, but becomes thickened, inflamed and tender. The main symptom is persistent headaches and great sensitivity of the scalp which may be so severe that the patient cannot bear even to wash their hair. The pain is worse on waking in the morning, and is sometimes accompanied by problems with vision such as diplopia or blurring. For it is not only the temporal artery which is involved, and other arteries may inflame and become blocked, particularly the ophthalmic artery supplying the eye and this may even lead to blindness unless it is urgently treated.

There is a close association between this disease and *polymyalgia rheumatica*, both occurring exclusively in elderly people and either coexisting or leading from one to the other. Polymyalgia is, as the name suggests, characterised by aching of the muscles particularly of the pelvis and shoulders, and there is often weight loss, fever and depression, signifying a generalised disorder. The erythrocyte sedimentation rate (ESR) (see glossary) is invariably raised and this gives useful support to the diagnosis. It is interesting that both the above conditions are associated with the presence of HLA DR4.

THE VEINS

These are more than just collecting channels, they form a reservoir which contains over half the blood in circulation, flowing gently under a low pressure. This predisposes them to thrombosis, especially when they are subjected to compression or stagnation. Because their walls are relatively thin, wherever back pressure on a vein happens it is likely to dilate and form a varix or several *varices* (L = bubble). Varices occur most often in the legs, where gravity has the greatest affect, and also at the anal margin (*haemorrhoids*), the lower end of the oesophagus (*oesophageal varices*) and in the scrotum or labia (*varicocele*).

VARICOSE VEINS

These are dilated, tortuous, superficial veins in the legs, either the *short saphenous vein* on the outer aspect or more commonly the *long saphenous vein* which runs from ankle to groin on the inner aspect (Gr. saphenous = outstanding). they are accompanied early on by cramps and itching, later by aching and heaviness particularly after standing and finally by such complications as ulceration and inflammation (*phlebitis*).

In most cases varicose veins arise because of an inherited defect of the valves of the legs, but the pressure from a pregnancy or occupations involving standing for long periods also predispose, as does damage to the valves from thrombophlebitis. Once a valve is damaged, the one below it is subjected to an even greater strain and this will also fail, until eventually the greatest pressure is exerted at the ankle. Here blood will leak out of the vessel and stain the skin, causing the irritation and dryness of *varicose eczema*, with eventual excoriation and infection. The skin may become devitalised and oedematous, finally breaking down as a *varicose ulcer* which may take many months to heal.

Although ulcers around the ankle are usually of varicose origin, they also arise in a number of other conditions, the main ones being *diabetes, intermittent claudication* and *rheumatoid arthritis*. African or West Indian patients with *sickle cell anaemia* are also prone to leg ulceration.

Apart from ulcerating, varicose veins may on occasions rupture and the resulting haemorrhage can become quite alarming. It may be controlled by elevating the leg and compressing the vein with a finger until the bleeding ceases, then bandaging firmly with a crepe bandage. If a varicose vein becomes acutely red, tender and inflamed then the patient is probably developing phlebitis, or more accurately *thrombophlebitis*, for usually the vein becomes thrombosed early on. Although painful, the condition is restricted to the superficial veins as a rule, and does not give rise to emboli in the circulation which normally come from the deep veins of the calf.

Phlebitis may arise in other veins in the body such as the brachial vein in the axilla, either as a result of local trauma – e.g. using a crutch – or as part of a general condition called *thrombophlebitis migrans*. In this unusual condition the phlebitis migrates to other areas of the body and causes an inflamed, tender cord where the vein has clotted. It may be the first sign of an underlying cancer, especially in the pancreas, and is thought to be the result of abnormal clotting mechanisms being initiated by the tumour.

DEEP VEIN THROMBOSIS (DVT)

This is a situation where the blood clots within one of the deep veins of the calf or pelvis, usually because the flow has become rather sluggish, the blood has become dehydrated or trauma has occurred in the area. Such events occur after abdominal surgery, heart attacks and childbirth, especially if the patient is confined to bed as the normal pumping effect of the muscles cannot stimulate the flow in the legs. In other cases the cause is an increased tendency for the blood to clot, either because of abnormal proteins present in certain cancers (see above) or due to drugs such as oestrogens (present in only very small quantities in contraceptive pills now, but sometimes use to treat tumours of the prostate and breast).

The patient usually (but not always) experiences some aching in the calf which may swell slightly. They may also be a little feverish and feel unwell. However, in many cases there are no symptoms and the diagnosis is not made until complications set in. The most alarming sequel to a deep venous thrombosis is that a piece breaks off and travels as an embolus up the inferior vena cava to the right side of the heart and thence to the lungs. Here it blocks the arteriole in which it comes to rest, causing ischaemia and quite possibly infarction of a segment of lung.

This **pulmonary embolus** as it is termed is one of the main causes of sudden death after an operation and the most vulnerable time is about one week postoperatively. If the embolus is large enough it is often immediately preceded by a desire to empty the bowels because of the stimulation of the vagus nerve as the embolus traverses the inferior vena cava, hence many of these patients are found collapsed in the toilet (one reason why hospital toilets have no locks).

If an *infarction* of the lung occurs there will be a sharp *pleuritic pain* and some *difficulty breathing*, sometimes followed by a slight *haemoptysis* a while later. Occasionally the DVT itself is symptomless and there are merely recurrent episodes of dyspnoea, wheeze and faintness which can go on for months until the patient develops pulmonary hypertension as the pulmonary tree is progressively blocked by emboli.

CHAPTER ELEVEN

LUNGS: DISORDERS OF BREATHING

Our lungs are in constant contact with the air, so much so that they might almost be thought of as being outside the body, yet they are extremely delicate organs and rely for their protection on the mechanisms of the upper part of the respiratory tract where the air is warmed, humidified and purified. It is therefore this area which is likely to become damaged by pollution or infected by bacteria and viruses to cause what are known as *upper respiratory tract infections* or URTI's and in turn this may lead to catarrh. The reaction of any mucus membrane to stimulation is to exude mucus to protect itself. Unfortunately the nasal passages are somewhat tortuous and narrow and may contain obstructions such as polyps and this prevents the free drainage of the catarrh which remains to cause a stuffy nose, sinusitis, earache or a chronic cough.

UPPER RESPIRATORY TRACT INFECTIONS

The common cold (coryza) is a pattern of symptoms associated with numerous different viruses, for well over 100 viruses cause cold symptoms and each must be experienced to develop some degree of immunity. Hence childhood is so often a period featuring nasal obstruction and discharge, sore throat and repeated coughs which last about 7–10 days. During a typical episode the mucus is clear to begin with but then becomes yellow or green with bacterial infection by about the third day. The main complications are otitis media in children, sinusitis in adults and hypostatic bronchopneumonia in the elderly or bedfast.

Laryngitis may be an accompaniment to a cold or may occur alone, especially in children, when it appears as *croup*. Adults developing laryngitis may lose their voice (aphonia) or complain of hoarseness, and usually recover within a day or two. Chronic hoarseness is likely to be due to inflammation of the cords from smoking, overuse of the voice or allergy. Occasionally it may be from swelling of the vocal cords which occurs in myxoedema, or from a tumour or nodule. On occasions the throat has the sensation of a lump in the region of the larynx although no swelling is palpable, and this is often the result of unexpressed grief being choked back and may go under the name of a *globus hystericus*.

Sinusitis is a condition mainly of adults and teenagers, as childrens' sinuses do not develop fully until puberty. Acute sinusitis follows either a blockage of the opening by a cold or allergy, or from diving. There is pain and tenderness over the sinus involved, either above the eyes in frontal sinusitis or beside the nostrils and in the upper teeth, which characteristically feel long, in maxillary sinusitis. The sphenoid and ethmoid sinuses are further back and give less trouble.

Chronic sinusitis may follow a physical obstruction such as a *deviated septum* or *polyp* which prevent free drainage, and these polyps are seen mostly in those with allergic rhinitis. The sinus fills with fluid and causes a *postnasal drip* with chronic catarrh and a persistant cough, and the fluid level within it may be seen by transilluminating the sinus through the mouth in a dark room using a bright torch.

Tonsillitis is often attributable to bacteria, especially streptococci, but some cases involve viruses, either an adenovirus infection or glandular

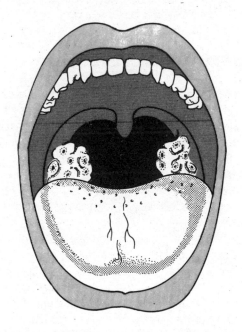

FIGURE 11.1   *Tonsillitis*

fever. The onset is sudden, with sore throat, fever, swollen tonsillar glands and malaise. The tonsils themselves are swollen and red, with pus or exudate visible in the crypts, and may go on to form an abscess known as a *quinsy* (peritonsillar abscess). Prior to the last war such symptoms were always a grave source of concern as they frequently indicated diphtheria, but this disease with its thick, white membrane adherent to the tonsils and toxic effect on the heart and nervous system is an extreme rarity nowadays.

Epiglottitis is a condition which is not common though serious when it appears, and is usually found in small children. It may initially be mistaken for croup, but the child is more severely ill and develops *stridor* or noisy breathing due to the obstruction of the swollen epiglottis which blocks the larynx. A particular strain of the bacterium Haemophilus is the usual cause.

Epistaxes or nose-bleeds are usually traumatic or spontaneous in origin and generally arise from the front of the nose on the septum, where they can be controlled by firm pressure between finger and thumb for at least five minutes continuously. Occasionally they are due to hypertension or even very rarely a bleeding disorder such as leukaemia or thrombocytopaenia. If they cannot be halted by pressure then the patient may need to have the nose packed with ribbon gauze.

ACUTE LUNG INFECTIONS

These normally follow the downward spread of a URTI into the lungs or the irritation of the trachea and bronchi by dust or chemicals, damp or cold. *Tracheitis* is a sore, scratchy retrosternal pain with only a little sputum unless it extends down into the bronchi as *acute bronchitis*, when there will be some wheeze with thick, yellow sputum and occasionally slight haemoptysis (coughing blood). The main risk is to babies, in whom the extension of the infection into the smaller bronchi, sometimes called *bronchiolitis*, has consequences similar to pneumonia and is one possible cause of cot death.

Influenza is a viral infection which gains its name from the fact that it was once thought to be under the influence of the stars which explained its periodic outbreaks as worldwide pandemics in which large numbers died of influenzal pneumonia. The most dramatic of these was the outbreak of 1918 when 20 million are said to have died, and more recently minor ones spread from Asia in 1957 and Hong Kong in 1968. There are three types of influenza virus, named A, B and C, of which only the first involves serious illness. However, type A is able to mutate and replace itself with a new 'subtype' every few years and this may infect birds as well as humans, which carry it far and wide.

The symptoms of 'flu are well known; there is a very brief incubation period of 2–3 days, then fever and muscle pains, followed usually by a dry cough and burning pains in the trachea. If the person is a smoker or elderly or suffers from chronic lung disease, then there is a real risk of secondary pneumonia following in the next day or two and causing severe shortness of breath. If the flu virus is of a very virulent strain then this may lead to a viral pneumonia, with copious blood-stained sputum and rapid death even in someone who was in good previous health.

PNEUMONIA

Acute lobar pneumonia, sometimes called *pneumococcal pneumonia* after the organism involved, is seen less often now but classically occurs in previously healthy young adults who suddenly contract it after being chilled. They develop a high fever with a flushed, dry skin and uncontrollable shivering (rigors), sometimes with a herpes lesion on the mouth. There is aching and malaise followed by a cough with viscid sputum and later a little rust-coloured haemoptysis and even cyanosis. Respiration is rapid and shallow and often painful as the pleura is usually involved and leads to sharp, stabbing pains on breathing. In the untreated case the symptoms increase until they reach a 'crisis phase' at the end of a week or so, when they either make a dramatic recovery or die. One or more lobes of the lung are affected by the pneumococcus, and there is congestion and *consolidation* of the tissue, and sometimes spread of the organism throughout the body as septicaemia. If recovery is incomplete a *lung abscess* may remain in the lobe, or fluid may leak into the pleural space and cause a *pleural effusion.*

Atypical pneumonia is the name given to the more commonly met condition of today, as the symptoms come on more slowly and are more variable depending on which of the different organisms is involved. These are either viruses, chlamydia (such as those caught from birds in psittacosis), mycoplasma or the Legionella bacillus of *Legionnaire's disease.* Although most are less virulent than lobar pneumonia, some, including Legionnaire's disease, have a significant mortality, and are more widespread than has been hitherto realised. The latter is a disease of especially the elderly and is more than just a pneumonia, for it involves the nervous system and digestive tract and may cause confusion, hallucinations and diarrhoea.

Another form of infection of the lungs, occurring especially in the elderly and the debilitated, is **bronchopneumonia**. This may be due to a variety of organisms which are able to invade because of the lowered resistance of the body and the poor circulation through the lungs. The base of the lungs and the bronchi become slowly infected and collapse, leading to stupor, confusion and eventually peaceful death, so bronchopneumonia is often seen as the terminal even of many chronic diseases. It may be a sequel to such things as heart failure, cancer or chronic bronchitis, and a similar form of pneumonia is seen after the aspiration of vomit through epilepsy, alcohol or drug abuse.

CHRONIC LUNG INFECTIONS

Any health worker in the industrial cities of the Midlands and North of England will have encountered **chronic bronchitis** or the 'English disease' as it is known. Although less common since the Clean Air Act of 1956, it still accounts for 30–40,000 deaths per annum with many more of its victims 'respiratory cripples', bound to their homes if not their beds by extreme breathlessness. Air pollution, dust, cigarette smoke and social factors combine to cause repeated attacks of acute bronchitis, especially in men, during the course of which the cilia are damaged so that eventually they cease to evacuate the debris which builds up and leads to a permanent irritation of the mucosal cells. These swell and pour out mucus which is coughed up each morning – the smoker's waking cough – and periodically become infected, causing still further damage and narrowing of the bronchioles. This leads to wheezing and sometimes to *emphysema*, the destruction of the partition walls of the alveoli and hence loss of the surface area of the lungs across which oxygen and carbon dioxide are transferred.

Either the bronchitis with its cough, wheeze and occasional haemoptysis, or else emphysema with its breathlessness is eventually likely to predominate in different individuals, and one of two clinical pictures will emerge. In the bronchitic the carbon dioxide cannot escape (it is more difficult to exhale than to inhale completely) and so is retained in the blood and causes central cyanosis which leads to drowsiness and a characteristic sluggish, Pickwickian appearance named the 'blue bloater'. The bloatedness is due in part at least to the oedema of the tissues which results from a degree of cor pulmonale (q.v.) common in this syndrome.

If **emphysema** predominates then ventilation (the movement of gas to and from the alveoli) is not a problem, but in order to transfer sufficient oxygen across his reduced alveolar area the patient must breathe more rapidly, and puffs rather than wheezes, usually blowing out his cheeks and holding his chest overinflated like a barrel. Cyanosis is not usually a problem because carbon dioxide can diffuse much more quickly than oxygen and readily escape, so they remain a healthy pink colour and are consequently known as 'pink puffers', but are usually extremely thin

125

perhaps owing to the amount of energy expended on breathing. Some cases of emphysema are familial and are caused by a deficiency of the enzyme antitrypsin which normally plays a protective role, but this is probably only relevant in those who smoke.

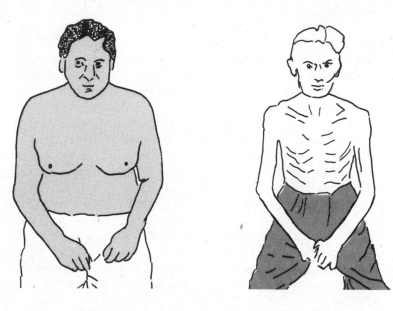

FIGURE 11.2   *A. Chronic bronchitis and B. Emphysema*

Bronchiectasis, like emphysema, is a destruction of tissue, but in this case involves the walls of the bronchi which dilate (Gr. ectasis = spread out). The pathological change which precedes and causes bronchiectasis is the occlusion of the small bronchi by secretions, coming from such diseases as *whooping cough, pneumonia* and *TB* especially during childhood. The lung tissue beyond the blockage collapses and the air is absorbed, a condition called *atelectasis* (Gr. atalos = delicate), and this shrinkage causes traction on the delicate walls of the infected bronchi which never regain their original shape but remain as dilated reservoirs of infection in different parts of the lung.

Thus arises the typical symptoms of cough with *profuse purulent sputum* and commonly *haemoptysis*, with loud rattling *crepitations* in the chest and eventually clubbing of the fingers (see below). Each morning at least the patient will require postural drainage by having someone assist

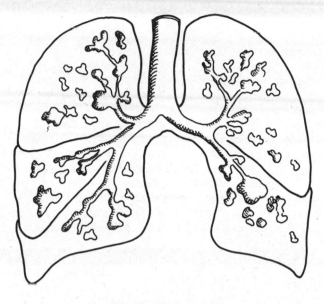

FIGURE 11.3   *Bronchiectasis*

loosen the sputum by smartly drubbing him on the back, when large quantities of often foul sputum will be coughed up. Sometimes the frontal sinuses are also chronically infected in this condition.

Cystic fibrosis gives rise to symptoms in children somewhat similar to those of bronchiectasis, but is a congenital disorder of the mucus produced in the glands of the pancreas and the bronchi. Owing to an enzyme defect this results in the mucus being much thicker than normal (hence the alternative name of '*mucoviscidosis*'), which leads to blockage of both the bronchioles and the pancreatic duct with both pumonary and digestive consequences. The physical signs and symptoms in the chest are mainly those of cough and breathlessness but with the addition of wheezing and weight loss, and usually start at an early age. Cystic fibrosis is the commonest congenital condition in the West and occurs in about 1 in 2000 births, but may vary in severity and the mildest cases remain undiagnosed as asthma or just 'chestiness' in a growing child. The diagnosis is established by measuring the concentration of salt in the sweat which is always raised, but as yet no test is available to discern carriers of the gene. In a badly affected child there are frequent severe chest infections and only half will live beyond the age of 20.

TABLE 11.1 Possible causes of cough in children

Condition	Pointers
Upper respiratory infection	Fever, sudden onset
Post-nasal drip	Chronic catarrh, sleeps through
Croup	Typical bark, sudden onset, under 3 yrs
Hay fever	Eyes itchy, no fever
Bronchitis	Fever, rattling breathing, crepitations
Pneumonia	High fever, rapid breathing, possibly cyanosis
Asthma	No fever, eczema, worst nights, probably wheeze
Pertussis	Fever, typical sound, paroxysms, vomiting
Inhaled foreign body	Abrupt onset, choking, blue
Epiglottitis	Fever, stridor, cyanosis, enlarged epiglottis
Cystic fibrosis	Chronic, weight loss, diarrhoea, repeated infns.

TABLE 11.2 Possible causes of cough in adults

Condition	Pointers
Upper respiratory infection	Fever, coryzal symptoms, blocked nose
Sinusitis	Sinus pain, catarrh
Laryngitis	Hoarse voice, no sputum
Influenza	Fever, myalgia, contact
Tracheitis	Dry cough, scratchy pain behind sternum
Acute bronchitis	Productive cough, sudden onset, inhaled dust
Pneumonia*	Sudden onset, rigors, high fever, pleurisy
Tuberculosis*	Night sweats, weight loss
Chronic bronchitis	Worse mornings, profuse sputum
Pulmonary embolus*	Sudden onset, sharp chest pain, breathlessness
Congestive heart failure	Breathlessness on exercise, basal crepitations
Cardiac asthma*	Worse at night, wheezing, pink frothy sputum
Lung cancer*	Smoker, losing weight, pneumonia, clubbing
Bronchiectasis*	Profuse green/yellow sputum, worse mornings
Sarcoidosis	Wheeze, erythema nodosum

(* indicates haemoptysis may be present)

TUBERCULOSIS

Until recently the word itself was sufficient to alarm a whole generation who had experienced relatives struck down apparently indiscriminately by

LUNGS

'phthisis' or 'consumption' as it was known, and who were raised on the works of Hardy and Dickens with their dramatic descriptions of the inexorable progression of the disease. In fact TB was always a byproduct of the industrial revolution, affecting predominantly the young, the female and the poor, lurking especially in the damp alleyways of conurbations and the misty glens of the Western Isles. Today in this country TB is uncommon and usually seen in older men, often immigrants from the third world, and the once familiar sight of the mobile X-ray unit is no longer seen. Periodically outbreaks still occur, however, and often when least expected, so one must be suspicious of the persistent cough, the night sweats and the unexplained loss of weight which are the usual presenting features.

The bacillus involved in this condition, *Mycobacterium tuberculosis*, has a unique mode of action which leads to the peculiar characteristics of the disease and its pathology. Its usual port of entry is via droplet infection into the lungs, but on occasions it may be swallowed and arrive in the wall of the gut, most often from infected milk. Once inside the body it is ingested by the large *macrophages*, which are monocytes that have migrated out of the blood to the tissues, but although these can ingest the bacteria they cannot kill them so a stalemate arises with nodules or 'tubercles' (L. = lump) arising at the site of entry usually the lymph nodes of the hilum of the lung. These primary foci of infection become a battle-ground between the multiplying bacteria and their surrounding macrophages, and in their centre an area of debris or *caseation* (L. caseus = cheese) builds up. In most reasonably healthy individuals the bacilli are destroyed eventually and the caseous area gradually calcifies to leave a 'shadow' on the lung and a positive reaction to the tuberculin or *Mantoux* (Heaf) test (which consists of challenging the body by inoculation with antigens from the protein wall of the bacillus and seeing whether it reacts). Thus ends the *primary infection*, usually acquired in childhood and usually without any symptoms apart from a slight cough and febrile illness, certainly nothing to make one suspect a potentially lethal disease.

However, in those whose immune system is defective in some way on account of chronic diseases such as diabetes, drug dependency or even simply lack of food, there develops a *progressive primary infection* as the organism overwhelms the inadequate macrophage response, and moves into the blood stream to set up metastatic foci elsewhere in the body, particularly the bones, kidneys, joints, skin, pericardium or adrenals. If the caseating focus is near a large vessel and invades it, then so-called *miliary tuberculosis* may spread seedling tubercles (L. milia = millet) to all areas of the body, including the brain and meninges, a frequently fatal outcome.

129

On rare occasions the lymphatic glands in the neck become swollen with tubercular pus, and may discharge a cheesy material – the *scrofula* or 'King's evil', so called because it was reputedly alleviated by the royal touch!

More usual than a progressive primary infection is what is known as a *postprimary infection*, which occurs many years after the initial primary infection because the baciillus breaks out of the area and escapes control. This tends to be the type of case seen nowadays in older men, who reactivate an old focus and present with the typical symptoms of cough with haemoptysis, dyspnoea, fever with night sweats and loss of weight. The characteristic quality of the postprimary type of infection is that it tends to form large *cavities* in the lungs, particularly in the apex, and this is where the physical signs are often heard and what gives rise to the name of 'consumption'.

Children who have not been exposed to a primary infection, shown by a negative Mantoux or Heaf test, are theoretically at risk if in contact with an active case of TB. They may be offered immunisation with an attenuated form of the bacillus called BCG, after the two men who invented it (Bacillus Calmette-Guerin).

SARCOIDOSIS

This is a somewhat mysterious disease, involving as it does so many different organs but with the lungs almost always playing a leading role. For many years it was thought to be a variety of TB as it is histologically very similar, but neither organisms nor caseation have ever been seen. The hallmark of the disease is the *granuloma*, a collection of chronic inflammatory cells, macrophages in particular. The name arises from the fact that granulomas were originally thought to be tumours with a granular appearance, and they are common to many other chronic diseases, such as TB, syphilis and leprosy.

A typical acute case starts in a young adult, with fever, stiff joints (especially the knees and ankles), swollen glands and breathlessness with a slight cough. A chest X-ray will reveal that the mediastinal glands are enlarged and there is a diffuse mottling in the lungs where the granulomas are seen. The severity of the condition varies, but almost all cases resolve in 2–3 years without treatment, although steroids are given if more serious features are evident. These include involvement of the eyes (uveitis), the heart (cardiomyopathy) and the nervous system (nerve palsies and meningitis).

A common and inexplicable feature in the earlier stages of many cases is a tender, dark red discoloration of the calves known as *erythema nodosum*, looking rather like a series of bruises running down the shins. This skin disorder occurs as a result of other conditions as well, in particular streptococcal throat infections, rheumatic fever, TB and reactions to some drugs. It is a peculiar and significant symptom and if seen should be investigated further.

BRONCHIAL ASTHMA

Asthma is one of the most frequently seen and significant lung disorders today, occurring in about 1 person in 7 to some degree and responsible for over 2000 deaths annually. It is defined as a reversible (as compared to chronic bronchitis) narrowing of the bronchioles of the lung, and tends to cause recurrent attacks of breathing difficulty against a background of general wheezing. Broadly speaking there are two main types of asthma, extrinsic and intrinsic, as well as the acute wheezy chest seen in some people when they develop an attack of bronchitis or chesty cold.

Atopic or **extrinsic asthma** is the common type occurring in

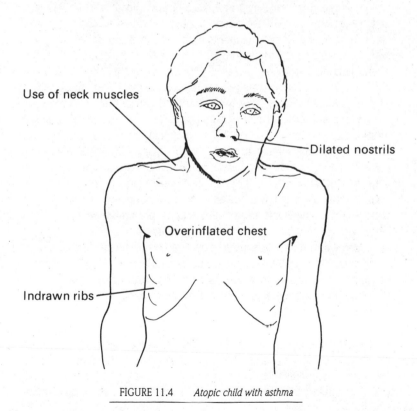

Use of neck muscles

Dilated nostrils

Overinflated chest

Indrawn ribs

FIGURE 11.4   *Atopic child with asthma*

children, especially boys, who have inherited an exaggerated or atopic (see chapter 2) response to a variety of allergens found in the environment. It seems that these children inherit the tendency to produce excessive quantities of antibodies in the form of immunoglobulins which renders them hypersensitive, so that the cells of the bronchioles react to the allergen violently and discharge chemicals such as histamine which make them constrict and swell up, so narrowing the airway. As well as bronchoconstriction, the effort to expel air in the act of expiration tends to collapse the bronchioles further, thus trapping air inside the alveoli which swell up like balloons. The upshot of this is the characteristic wheeze and prolonged, difficult exhalation seen in an acute attack, which may come on quite suddenly. The exhalation is prolonged because it is essentially a passive act accomplished by the elastic qualities of the lung, and the trapping of air in the overinflated chest gives it a barrel-shaped symmetry and limited movement of the ribs, which can be seen in severe chronic asthmatics.

The small bronchioles also produce mucus which eventually dries and plugs the air passages in a prolonged episode, leading to oxygen lack and cyanosis in a severe case. Most episodes of asthma occur at night and last 1–2 hours unless they are due to emotional causes or follow URTIs in which case they may be prolonged. If the attack continues for several hours without responding to reatment than it is termed 'status asthmaticus', and the risks are correspondingly increased. One of the most serious signs of this is the 'silent chest' when very little noise can be heard as the person breathes, for the simple reason that so little movement of air in the lungs is taking place. This is usually accompanied by a degree of cyanosis and demands most urgent treatment with oxygen. Many children have quite frequent episodes of asthma but between attacks the child may scarcely wheeze at all and may simply have a characteristic *dry cough*. This continuous cough without any mucus is often the first sign that a child is developing atopic asthma, and may be present for several months before any overt wheezing is noticed, especially during the night.

Atopic asthma can be provoked by a variety of stimuli, the usual ones being pollen grains, animal dander, moulds and, by far the most common, housedust. In addition there are some irritant substances which we all react to, such as sulphur dioxide and tobacco smoke which, while not allergenic, can stimulate an attack. Housedust consists largely of shed human skin, of which we all lose several pounds each year, and a microscopic-size insect, or more specifically spider, called the housedust mite feeds on these scales once they have been softened by yeasts. Dampness encourages the yeasts, and hence the housedust mites, and the latter accumulate in larger numbers in bedding, pillows (especially feather ones), carpets and furnishing, especially in modern warm houses.

It is actually the droppings of the mite which form the allergens which cause asthma, and the usual advice given is to vacuum the house thoroughly every day. However, if a standard vacuum cleaner is used the bag is porous enough to allow most of the droppings to pass through and be sprayed out into the air, exacerbating the problem, so it is important to invest in a modern microfilter type such as the Medivac. Furthermore, the bedrooms should be kept as cold as possible throughout the day to inhibit the mites from breeding, and as dry as possible, if necessary by using a dehumidifier, to discourage the yeasts. Before vacuuming the carpets and the furniture should be sprayed with a dilute solution of tannic acid which breaks down the proteins in the droppings and renders them less allergenic. Although this represents a considerable outlay in equipment, the long term dangers of asthma are serious and include pulmonary damage as well as postural and psychological changes.

Intrinsic asthma is the name given to that variety of asthma which emerges usually in later life and in which allergic stimuli play only a minor part. It is mostly seen in women, in whom attacks of asthma occur against a background of general wheeziness, and it is in this group that most fatalities occur. There is a high incidence of nasal polypi in such people which complicates breathing still further, and they are sometimes allergic to aspirin or NSAIDS which are liable to provoke a severe attack. Many chemicals used in the food industry can trigger a bout of asthma in those susceptible, especially tartrazine, benzoic acid and sulphites (used as a preservative), and in some people exercise itself can be a cause.

DRUGS AND ASTHMA

The orthodox treatment of asthma is based on three types of drugs which act in rather different ways. The most rapidly acting are those which have an effect on the sympathetic nerves which dilate the bronchi, an action which is performed in the body by adrenalin. For many years this was given by injection for asthma, but is extremely dangerous because of its tendency to overstimulate the heart and raise the blood pressure, and adrenalin-type aerosols were responsible for many deaths in the earliy 60s. Research indicated that the lungs responded to sympathetic stimulation in a rather different way from the alpha-receptors (as opposed to the beta-receptors of the heart). A drug which stimulates these alpha receptors is salbutamol (Ventolin), but if given orally can provoke a slight adrenalin-like response with irritability and hyperactivity in children, so it is usually given as an inhaled spray every four hours.

Because most asthma attacks are a result of inflammation and swelling of the mucosa of the bronchioles, as well as bronchoconstriction, cortisone and its derivative drugs are successful in suppressing this reaction and are sometimes used for severe asthma in tablet form. However, if given over a prolonged period, for more than three weeks, the side effects begin to mount up and difficulties of withdrawal are experienced, so it is usually taken as an aerosol spray in the form of beclomethasone (Becotide) when very small doses will suffice. Insufficient quantities of cortisone are absorbed to have an effect on the pituitary feedback mechanism so the safety margin is very wide, however, some notice local side-effects in the form of sore throats and occasionally thrush.

With a condition such as asthma it makes sense to prevent attacks rather than treating each separately, and this is what a third line of treatment attempts to do (Becotiode is also prophylactic to some extent). It was found that certain chrome salts prevented the reaction between the mast cells of the mucosa and the allergen, but these must be given as an inhaled powder continually for some days before an effect is noticeable. The substance, sodium chromoglycate (Intal), is taken 4 times daily and in many

TABLE 11.3	Possible causes of breathlessness
Condition	**Pointers**
Sudden Onset (minutes or hours)	
Asthma	Wheeze, recurrence, long expiration
Hyperventilation	Emotional factors, absence of ill health
Cardiac Asthma	Nocturnal onset, frothy sputum, pallor
Pneumonia	Pyrexia, rapid breathing, pain, signs
Pulmonary Embolus	Possible calf swelling, pain
Pneumothorax	Abrupt onset, fit person, signs in chest
Diabetic Ketosis	Sighing respiration, dry tongue, diabetic
Altitude Sickness	Sudden onset, headache, insomnia
Gradual Onset (weeks or months)	
Chronic Bronchitis	Long history, purulent sputum
Emphysema	Long history, barrel chest, weight loss
Heart Failure	Worse on exercise, cough, crepitations
Lung Cancer	Smoker, cough, weight loss, haemoptysis
Anaemia	Usually iron deficiency, occasionally B12
Pleural Effusion	Cancer, rheumatoid arthritis, pneumonia
Recurrent Pulmonary Embolus	Often silent, previous operation or labour
Tuberculosis	Weight loss
Pulmonary Fibrosis	

will reduce the incidence of attacks, especially if they are related to exercise.

LUNG CANCER

Bronchial carcinoma, arising from the cells lining the small bronchi, is by far the commonest cause of cancer among men and has increased thirtyfold since the beginning of the century and is now responsible for about one death in every 20, although it is at last levelling off. Although women are much less likely to contract it, current smoking patterns among girls indicate that it will have overtaken breast cancer to reach the number one spot within the next few years. Because our bronchial mucosa is continually in contact with the environment it acts as a kind of 'pollution meter' for such substances as tars, soot, hydrocarbons and many other carcinogens, which means that the inhalation of others' tobacco smoke also increases our risk substantially. Depending on the amount smoked and the number of years of exposure, mutations of the cells result which eventually lead to malignant change.

The type of cancer and its rate of growth depends on its similarity to its parent cell, in other words the degree to which it has specialised or *differentiated* from a primitive cell. A cancerous cell which is a very crude imitation of its original tissue, i.e. is *undifferentiated*, tends to have few controls over its growth and is therefore highly malignant. Such cancers make up about half the cases and are sometimes termed 'oat-cell' carcinomas after their resemblance to an ear of the grain on the stalk.

Between the inception of a cancer and the appearance of symptoms lies a period of 2–3 years, during which time the tumour is growing locally, but at some point vessels and lymphatics are likely to be invaded and convey the malignant cells to a distant site in the form of a *metastasis*. The first evidence of anything amiss may therefore be from a symptom far removed from the area, such as an epileptic fit or a fracture, for lung cancer tends to spread to the *brain, bones, liver* and *adrenal glands*. Very often the first metastasis appears in the lymphatic tissues as a swollen lymph gland in the mediastinum first seen on X-ray.

A 'typical' case of bronchial carcinoma would be a middle-aged man who smokes and gradually loses weight and feels unwell over a period of about six weeks, experiences a persistent and irritating cough and becomes a little breathless. Eventually he might experience some dull pain in the chest and cough up a little blood. When the tumour has enlarged enough to block the bronchus completely the lung beyond it will collapse (*atalectasis*) and become infected, leading to a fever and sudden worsening of symptoms. Later one of a number of different signs may appear, especially:

135

– *pleural effusion.* If the tumour lies in the outer part of the lung then its spread will take it to the pleura which reacts by secreting bloodstained fluid into the pleural cavity. This is always painful and accounts for much of the pain felt by patients with this disease, moreover the effusion may become infected and form an *empyema*, a collection of pus in the pleural cavity (this occasionally occurs after pneumonia also). Further, the pericardium itself may be invaded and lead to pericarditis.

– *superior vena cava syndrome* occurs when the enlarging growth compresses the thin-walled superior vena cava in the mediastinum and obstructs the blood returning to the heart, causing swelling and plethora of the neck and shoulders.

– *Horner's syndrome* (see chapter 19).

– *clubbing of the fingers*, a strange and inexplicable condition of the fingernails and to a lesser extent the toes, whereby the nails become increasingly curved and eventually swell like a drumstick. It is found in lung disorders such as TB, bronchiectasis, emphysema and alveolitis, in congenital heart disease and in cirrhosis, Crohn's disease and ulcerative colitis.

– *hoarseness* due to damage to the recurrent laryngeal nerve.

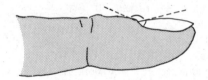

Normal nail, showing angle between nail and bed

Early clubbing, angle lost

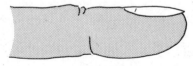

Late clubbing, nail bed swollen

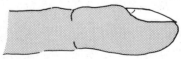

FIGURE 11.5   *Normal nail, early and advanced clubbing*

RESPIRATORY FAILURE

Just as heart failure is the inability to pump blood, so respiratory failure is the inability to oxygenate it, and this may happen for two reasons. Firstly because the *ventilation* of the lungs, that is the movement of air in and out, is inadequate because of obstruction in some form or another – *'obstructive airways disease'*, and this applies to any disorder where the bronchi are narrowed. But a second problem may also occur, that of *diffusion* across the alveolar membrane, and this is reduced when the membrane is thickened for any reason.

When ventilation is diminished, as happens in asthma and chronic bronchitis, the oxygen is unable to enter and the patient exhibits symptoms of *hypoxia* – confusion, dizziness, drowsiness and weakness, similar to those seen in altitude sickness where the oxygen content of the air is very low. This is the first indication that they are developing a dangerous state and require oxygen quickly. At the same time CO_2 is retained in the alveoli as it cannot escape, and will eventually build up in the blood leading to a bluish tinge – *'central cyanosis'*. By the time this has happened there will be quite a severe degree of obstruction to the airways and treatment is urgent. Of course the distinction must be made between central cyanosis due to respiratory failure and peripheral cyanosis due to sluggishness of the blood in the periphery such as occurs on the lips and skin of those who are thoroughly chilled.

Impairment of diffusion of gas across the alveolar membrane is usually limited to oxygen alone, as CO_2 can move across much more easily and quickly. Therefore cyanosis seldom appears in those who suffer from disease of their alveoli, and they are breathless without being cyanosed. As well as the destruction of the alveoli in emphysema already mentioned, a similar situation arises due to thickening of the membrane, either from fibrosis or inflammation from allergy – 'allergic alveolitis'. The latter condition is a result of inhaling moulds as in farmers lung (hay), bird fancier's lung (bird droppings) etc. Pulmonary fibrosis occurs in connective tissue diseases such as rheumatoid arthritis, systemic lupus erythematosis and sarcoidosis, as well as in industrial lung disease caused by the inhalation of particles and chemicals. These particles generate a reaction in the alveoli and cause them to atrophy and thicken as tiny scars, leading to gross dyspnoea and clubbing of the fingers but no cyanosis. The main problem is that the fibrosis also extends to involve the lung capillaries and leads to great strain on the right ventricle which eventually fails from cor pulmonale.

THE PLEURA

These membranes surrounding the lungs contain a large number of pain receptors and their stimulation provokes a typically sharp, stabbing pain which is exacerbated especially by deep breathing. Because the pleura also cover the diaphragm which is innervated by the phrenic nerve, stimulation of this area may be felt as a pain referred to the shoulder.

Pleurisy is an extremely painful condition of the pleura which is normally the result of an acute infection of the underlying lung such as pneumonia, TB or some other lung condition. The most common non-infective causes are pulmonary embolus, a spreading carcinoma of the bronchus or occasionally rheumatoid arthritis. As well as giving rise to pains, the pleural membrane reacts by secreting fibrin which roughens the surface and may cause a *pleural rub* with each inspiration, audible with a stethoscope and not unlike a hinge which needs oiling. In some cases quantities of clear fluid are poured into the pleural space as a *pleural effusion*, and the lung is slowly compressed. If the fluid later becomes infected it changes to pus and an *empyema* is said to have occurred.

One specific cause of pleuritic-type pain is an infection by the

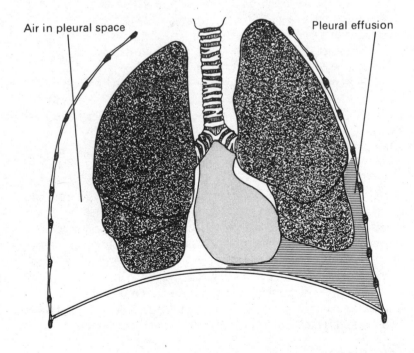

Air in pleural space   Pleural effusion

FIGURE 11.6   *Pneumothorax and pleural effusion*

Coxsackie B virus known as *Bornholm disease* after the island on which the first known outbreak occurred. Although the pain is pleuritic in character it is actually the underlying muscles of the chest wall which are mostly involved, hence the alternative name of 'epidemic myalgia'. The first symptoms are a fever and sore throat, followed a day or two later by the pains which may linger on for a week or more but will eventually clear without complications.

Pneumothorax is another condition involving the pleura and is caused by the rupture of a weak area of the outer wall of the lung, usually at the apex, which allows air to pass through into the thoracic cavity – the pneumothorax. The weakness is sometimes the result of chronic obstructive airways disease or emphysema, but may occur spontaneously in young adults, especially men who tend to be tall and thin. They experience a sudden pain in the side of the chest, perhaps while straining at something, followed by breathlessness as the lungs are compressed by the escaping air, but this often diminishes within half an hour or so as the other lung takes over and may even resolve spontaneously. If necessary the air can be drained out of the thorax via a one-way valve, when the pleura usually heals itself. However, spontaneous pneumothorax is likely to recur periodically and sometimes eventually requires an operation to seal the potential holes.

CHAPTER TWELVE

MOUTH & STOMACH: DISORDERS OF DIGESTION

*T*he mouth sustains a complex population of bacteria which maintains a stable ecology and under normal circumstances prevents pathogenic organisms from invading. This ecology is also dependent on the general nutritional state of the individual and is reflected in the more subtle changes which are seen on the tongue. Deficiencies of the B complex vitamins, iron and other elements can be observed by examining the tongue, which has been raised to a subtle art in Chinese tongue diagnosis. A disturbance in the balance is responsible for furring of the tongue or halitosis (bad breath), but a more severe infection may occur after the resident population has been decimated by antibiotics, especially the broad-spectrum ones like tetracyclene, or else the normal function of the immune system impaired by drugs such as cortisone or diseases such as leukaemia, aplastic anaemia or AIDS. The resulting inflammation of the mouth is known as *stomatitis*, or *glossitis* if the tongue is predominantly involved. Inflammation of the lip is called a *cheilitis* or *cheilosis*.

Candida (monilia, thrush) is a common type of stomatitis, so-called because of its resemblance to the speckled appearance of a thrush's breast, and is commonly seen on the cheek, tongue and palate of babies and the elderly or debilitated. Babies may contract the condition from the mother during birth, while the elderly sometimes develop chronic fissures at the corners of the mouth − 'angular cheilitis'. The area surrounding the thrush is red and sore, and the deposit cannot be scraped off, which distinguishes it from milk in young babies. Sometimes the oseophagus is involved, and after a course of antibiotics some people notice some difficulty in swallowing for a few days.

Candida may also be found sometimes in the intestines, especially if there is diabetes present or the person has been on cortisone or broad spectrum antibiotics. Because candida is a yeast, its spores are found everywhere and only a healthy gut is able to prevent colonisation, so intestinal candidasis may reflect an underfunctioning immune system. The consequences of this are that certain foodstuffs, and even candida itself, may penetrate into the bloodstream and lead to sensitivity reactions in the body. These can manifest in a variety of ways, ranging from headaches and depression to cystitis and dyspepsia.

Stomatitis which actually leads to ulcers may be caused by *herpes simplex* or by *aphthous ulceration* (Gr. apto=set on fire), when usually the tongue or inside of the cheek or lip is involved. Aphthae occur in crops as shallow, painful ulcers with a white rim and last for several days, appearing in those who are generally below par or suffer from food sensitivity or ulcerative colitis. Herpes simplex is a virus of the herpes family (see chapter 3) and attacks either the mouth and lips (HS1 or herpes labialis) or the genitalia (HS2 or herpes genitalis), producing a blister which rapidly ulcerates and crusts over. The first attack occurs in childhood in most people, and may involve a wide area of the gums and mouth – *herpetic stomatitis* – so the child is quite ill and feverish. Subsequent attacks, when the virus re-emerges from its dormant state, occur during periods of stress or exposure to the sun and wind and usually involve the lips (cold sore).

Leukoplakia is a chronic, premalignant condition involving the side of the tongue or the inside of the cheek, and appears as a thickened white plaque of tissue often at the site of continuous abrasion by such things as badly fitting dentures or a pipe. Most cases will eventually go on to become cancerous after a number of months or years, so should not be ignored.

Most cases of glossitis are due to a deficiency of *iron* or one of the *B vitamins*, especially B2 (Riboflavin), B12 or nicotinic acid. The moist velvety appearance is lost and the tongue appears smooth, sore and red or purple with atrophy of the papillae. The 'geographical tongue' is so-called because the loss of papillae is partial, leading to the resemblance to a map, but has no pathological significance. Heavy furring of the tongue may result from smoking or dietary disorders, and an extreme case is the 'black hairy tongue' which may relate to previous antibiotics. The 'strawberry tongue' of scarlet fever is described in chapter 3.

Gingivitis, or periodontitis as it is called when an area immediately surrounding the teeth is involved, is usually a result of poor dental hygiene. Organisms, especially Vincent's spirochaete, invade the tissue and cause leakage of pus (*pyorrhoea*) and even ulceration if neglected. Swelling of the gums may be a side-effect of phenytoin (Epanutin) therapy for epilepsy, and very rarely gum disease is due to vitamin C deficiency or scurvy.

The salivary glands seldom cause trouble unless there is much sepsis in the mouth, when the parotid particularly may inflame to cause a parotitis with a red, tender swelling. *Mumps* is a mild form of parotitis. In some cases of Parkinsonism there is an increase in salivation from the glands which may be troublesome, while in middle-aged women in particular the opposite may happen and the secretions from the salivary glands dry up, a condition known as *Sjogren's syndrome* and associated with drying of the joints and arthritis, sometimes also with absence of tears and gritty eyes. Another reason why one salivary gland may swell intermittently is the presence of a stone in the duct preventing the exit of saliva. The symptom will manifest mostly during meal times, and a *calculus* may be felt in the duct.

THE OESOPHAGUS

The only function of the oesophagus is to transport food through the thorax to the stomach, and as it is the narrowest part of the alimentary canal we can see why the main symptom of disease here is difficulty swallowing (*dysphagia*).

A *pharyngeal pouch* or diverticulum may appear in middle-age at the junction of the pharynx and the oesophagus where there is an area of potential weakness, and the patient will develop regurgitation of food. A swelling in the neck may be visible which will empty noisily under pressure, and eventually there will be some dysphagia at the top of the oesophagus. This is in contrast to that sometimes felt at the lower end in those who develop spasm of the cardiac sphincter – cardiospasm or *achalasia* (Gr. chaleo = to loosen). This occurs mostly in middle-aged women, in whom the nerve cells of the oesophageal plexus atrophy so that there is gradual failure of relaxation of the sphincter and corresponding hesitation in the food entering the stomach. Both of the above are uncommon causes of dysphagia, more frequently it is caused by a hiatus hernia, a foreign body of some kind or a carcinoma.

Hiatus hernia and the accompanying reflux of acid (*reflux oesophagitis*) is probably the commonest cause of oesophageal problems, and consists of herniation of the upper part of the stomach through a hiatus or gap in the diaphragm which may be unnaturally weak or subject to exceptional pressure from obesity, pregnancy etc. This may be symptomless in some people but in others leads to disruption of the cardiac sphincter with corresponding reflux of acid from the stomach which may regurgitate into the mouth and even spill over into the lungs and lead to persistent episodes of chest infection. Since the oesophagus is not designed to withstand acidity there is a painful sensation (heartburn) and sometimes ulceration of the mucous membrane of the lower oesophagus.

The reflux is worst when the patient stoops, lifts or lies down, especially after a big meal. Conversely loosening tight clothing, propping the head of the bed on bricks and taking alkaline fluids relieve the symptoms. Hiccoughs may sometimes be a problem due to stimulation of the diaphragm, and occasionally the hernia is so large that it actually compresses the lung and causes dyspnoea. Complications from a hiatus hernia arise from the ulceration of the oesophagus which oozes blood and may lead to anaemia if iron stores are deficient. Or it may heal with much scarring and fibrosis with a resulting stricture and dysphagia.

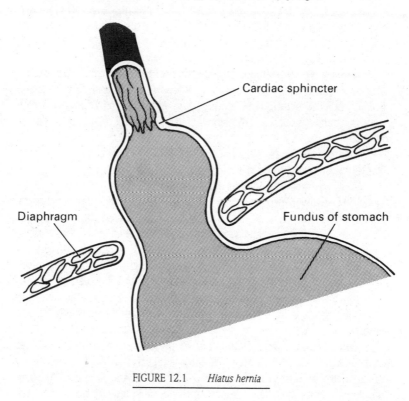

Cardiac sphincter

Diaphragm

Fundus of stomach

FIGURE 12.1   *Hiatus hernia*

Oesophageal cancer occurs mostly in elderly men, especially smokers, and has a poor prognosis as it rapidly ulcerates through the wall and spreads to other structures, so early diagnosis is important. The lower part of the oesophagus is where it tends to occur and where the dysphagia is noted, first for solids and then later for liquids also. It is extremely common in some parts of the world, especially China (owing to the high temperature at which food is swallowed and the high content of spices and moulds found in the diet) and Japan (where it has been associated with eating bracken fern).

THE STOMACH

The necessity of the stomach to secrete acid for digestion of proteins is also its main weakness should the resistance of the mucosal lining fail. If this happens then the result is gastritis which may progress to *peptic ulceration* and this may occur in the *stomach, oesophagus* or *duodenum*. The balance between the acid and the mucus protection is a delicate one, influenced by factors such as dental decay, diet, smoking, alcohol, the reflux of bile from the duodenum and particularly emotional stress which all play a part. Recently there has been evidence that gastritis and peptic ulcers are caused by an infection by bacteria of the Campylobacter species. This has been found in about 90% of duodenal ulcers and 75% of gastric ulcers, and the organism produces large quantities of ammonia which may neutralise the acid, although why this should lead to ulceration is unclear.

Gastric ulcers are ulcers of the lining of the stomach, often located on the lesser curvature near the pylorus (see figure 12.2). They are found particularly in men and women from economically and socially deprived areas, especially in Scotland and the North of England, and tend to be chronic and recur every few weeks as a flare-up in the continuous background of gnawing epigastric pain, especially after an alcoholic drink. The pain is also characteristically worse after eating, when acid is secreted, so the sufferers tend to avoid food and lose weight, and find relief from vomiting. Multiple tiny ulcers called *gastric erosions* are seen sometimes as side-effects of some drugs, particularly aspirin, cortisone and the NSAIDS which can lead to bleeding and melaena, especially in the elderly.

Duodenal ulcers on the other hand are seen mostly in younger men in high-pressured, stressful careers ('executive ulcers'), and in many cases there is an excessive secretion of acid by the stomach. Women are largely immune from these ulcers, possibly for hormonal reasons. The pain is identical in quality to that of a gastric ulcer but tends to be present several hours after a meal when the stomach is empty, sometimes waking the patient in the small hours of the morning as a 'hunger-pain'. Relief is usually sought by eating bland food or drinking milk, so they may put on weight and look surprisingly well-nourished.

Peptic ulcers may come and go quite quickly, resembling aphthous ulcers in this respect, but some run a prolonged course for months and

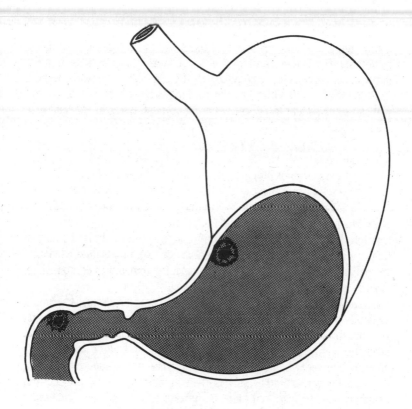

FIGURE 12.2   *Typical sites for gastric and duodenal ulcer*

even years. Some even develop complications, the main ones being as follows:

– *Bleeding.* This may be very heavy if an artery is eroded, and the stomach or duodenum fills with blood which may be vomited – (*haematemesis*). If the blood has been in the stomach for a while, the acid will oxidise it to a dark brown material with the appearance of coffee grounds. In some the blood first appears in the stools as tarry black *melaena* (Gr. melanos = black) which has a characteristic, rather pungent odour. Both haematemesis and melaena signify bleeding fairly high in the digestive tract, not necessarily from an ulcer. Other possibilities are from an *erosion* in the stomach, usually due to aspirin or similar drugs (see above), from a *stomach tumour* or from leaking *oesophageal varices* (see chapter 14).

– Perforation. Few ulcers are severe enough to penetrate into the peritoneal cavity, but occasionally one does, especially if the patient is taking steroids, and the result is that acid flows out and causes a chemical *peritonitis.* The first evidence of this is a sudden, excruciating pain in the upper abdomen which is aggravated by the slightest movement. Because the diaphragm is often involved the pain may be felt in the shoulders but will cause the patient to lie absolutely *motionless.* Even the bowels cease their peristalsis and the result is complete silence of the bowel sounds, later with distension as air finds its way into the peritoneum. After a few hours the patient is liable to become shocked and require an operation, when the perforation is plugged with a convenient piece of omentum.

– Stenosis. Narrowing of the pylorus or even the lower part of the stomach may occur in the case of an ulcer which has healed repeatedly with much scarring and fibrosis. If peristalsis is unable to urge food through, the stomach will dilate until it is two or three times its normal size, and then vomit up old food eaten one or two days before. Obviously the patient will lose weight rapidly and become thin and undernourished, so this situation is often mistaken for cancer.

Congenital pyloric stenosis, though unrelated to ulcers, is a similar situation occurring in some newborn babies who have a congenital hypertrophy of the pyloric muscle. The baby, usually a first-born male, begins to vomit its feeds and lose weight at the age of 3–4 weeks. The vomitus emerges with great force ('projectile vomiting') a short while after the feed is over, and the baby is then immediately hungry again and demands another feed, only for the process to be repeated. Sometimes peristalsis may be visible through the abdominal wall, and the enlarged sphincter felt on palpation. If the situation does not settle an operation to widen the pylorus may be required.

STOMACH CANCER

Gastric carcinoma has actually declined in Britain over the last 30 years but is still the most common form of cancer in both men and women after lung, breast and colon. In some countries, e.g. Japan and Portugal, the incidence is 2-3 times as high as in Britain and the US which suggests that dietary factors are involved, and the chief culprit is thought probably to be nitrate derivatives, some of which are highly carcinogenic. These take the form of nitrosamines which are derived through the combination of nitrites with amines in the food by gut organisms, and this reaction is blocked by vitamin C which thus has a protective effect.

Individuals with little or no acid in their stomachs (achlorhydria), a situation prevalent in pernicious anaemia and after gastrectomy, are at a much greater risk as the bacteria which perform the nitrosamine reaction are able to survive in the stomach. There is also a possibility that cimetidine, a drug much used to lower the acid content in the stomachs of ulcer patients, will have a similar effect. Moreover, we now have a situation where the quantities of nitrates used by modern farming as fertilizer are so great that the water table is becoming contaminated. Strangely, the incidence of cancer in the small intestine is extremely low, and no theory has adequately explained this. It may be that the very high turnover of cells which are continually being shed prevents abnormal tissue remaining long in the body, or perhaps that the secretions of the small bowel are so prolific that the potential carcinogens are diluted.

Most cases of stomach cancer arise in the region of the pylorus, and hence obstruct the outflow and lead to nausea and discomfort after food. This symptom occurring in a 50–60 year old should arouse suspicion, and enquiry will often reveal *anorexia, weight loss* and vague *dyspepsia*. Eventually there will be vomiting of food similar to the pyloric stenosis following a gastric ulcer, and indeed a gastric ulcer, though not a duodenal, may sometimes become malignant after a number of years. If the tumour is up at the cardiac end of the stomach, then the predominant symptom is likely to be dysphagia, and perhaps the appearance of a node in the supraclavicular area. A common accompanying feature is bleeding, which may pass unnoticed for a while until the patient becomes obviously pale and anaemic, by which time he may have metastatic spread to the lymph nodes and the liver, when jaundice is likely to ensue. The terminal picture is that of extreme weight loss (*cachexia*), pallor, jaundice and ascites containing malignant cells. The prognosis is unfortunately poor and only about 5% survive more than 5 years.

THE PANCREAS

This gland has two functions, the secretion of the hormones insulin and glucagon for the control of glucose metabolism, and the secretion of enzymes into the duodenum for digestion of fat, protein and carbohydrate. Failure of its first function of course produces diabetes mellitus, but fortunately this seldom affects enzyme production and digestion is not impaired. Less commonly the whole gland is affected by blockage, tumour or inflammation and the result is the passage of undigested fat in the stools – *steatorrhoea* (Gr. steatos = fat) and the inability to absorb nutrients from the small intestine – *malabsorption*.

Cystic fibrosis is the usual cause of blockage of the pancreatic ducts, and is due to an inherited defect in the glands of the body which produce mucus. It is the commonest genetic defect in Britain but extremely rare

147

among Asians and Africans. The glands secrete mucus which is much too viscid and blocks the ducts, because insufficient water is taken up by the gland. The result in the pancreas is that its enzymes are prevented from emerging into the duodenum and digestion does not take place adequately. The characteristic symptoms are thus those of excessive fat in the stools (*steatorrhoea*) and failure of the child to thrive. As the lungs are also involved in the condition there is often chestiness and wheezing with repeated respiratory infections. The severity of the condition depends largely on the degree of stickiness of the mucus, but in a severe case the child will require supplements of pancreatic enzymes with each meal and is likely to die prematurely. Another feature is that the sweat is extremely salty, and this is used as the basis of a test used to confirm the diagnosis.

Cancer of the pancreas is a less common tumour of the gut but notoriously difficult to diagnose as it may present in a variety of different ways. This may be as *jaundice*, owing to blockage of the common bile duct, as vague dyspeptic symptoms such as nausea, vomiting and anorexia, or as a dull pain in the upper abdomen often radiating through to the back, relieved by bending double. Sometimes there is an inexplicable fever, or phlebitis which moves around the body ('thrombophlebitis migrans'). It is thought that there is a possible link between the incidence of pancreatic carcinoma and a high consumption of coffee.

Pancreatitis is an inflammation of the pancreas and may be either acute or chronic in its onset. The acute type is caused by the pancreas suddenly digesting itself with its own proteolytic enzymes (Gr. pan = all; kreas = meat). The reason for this is not known, but there is usually a history of either *gallstones* or *alcoholism*, and in most cases reflux of bile up the pancreatic duct due to a malfunction of the sphincter of Oddi.

The pain is severe and located in the epigastrium, coming on quickly and radiating through to the back, but typically eased by leaning forward. The patient looks and is very ill and shocked (the mortality rate is about 50%) and may develop jaundice. The chronic type of pancreatitis consists of fibrosis of the gland following repeated acute attacks or simply damage by alcohol. The pain is less severe but recurrent, especially after alcohol, and the patient will begin to lose weight and may even become diabetic if the Islets of Langerhans are involved.

CHAPTER THIRTEEN

INTESTINES: DISORDERS OF ABSORPTION

SMALL INTESTINE

Because almost all the nutrients which enter the body are absorbed through the wall of the small intestine, the most significant consequence of disorders of this organ is *malabsorption*. One of the features of this is a dramatic loss of weight, and this is common to allergic, infective and inflammatory conditions and is accompanied by the passage of undigested food in the stools, especially fat, which is termed *steatorrhoea*. If peristalsis is also affected there will be accompanying colicky pains and diarrhoea, sometimes with bleeding.

Coeliac disease is the main allergic cause of malabsorption, and was first described in 1888 by Dr Gee of Gee's Linctus fame. His description was of infants who, soon after weaning, began to lose weight and pass frequent pale, bulky and offensive stools which floated on water. They were very miserable children with distended abdomens and emaciated

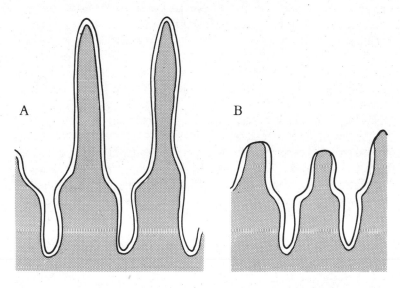

FIGURE 13.1   *A. Normal and B. Atrophic villi of coeliac disease*

limbs, later developing anaemia, bruising and dermatitis due to vitamin and iron deficiency. The condition occurred in about one child in 2000 and was generally fatal, but mysteriously disappeared in many countries for the duration of World War II, only to reappear again afterwards. At length it was realized that a protein called *gluten*, present in wheat, rye, barley and oats was responsible for the symptoms, and that by excluding these from the diet the child recovered.

Apparently these children were allergic to the gluten which caused the villi of the small intestine to atrophy in part and limit the absorptive power of the gut, so the alternative name for the condition is *gluten enteropathy*. The symptoms commenced soon after weaning with loss of weight, wind and a distended abdomen, offensive diarrhoea containing undigested food and eventually bruising due to a lack of vitamin K. A similar condition is found less frequently in adults, who develop the emaciation and anaemia but not necessarily the steatorrhoea, indeed they often become constipated at the onset of the condition which is known as *adult coeliac disease*. It may also be accompanied by an intractable itching and blistering of the skin.

Crohn's disease is a somewhat more mysterious condition whose aetiology is unknown, though some suspect an allergic basis here too. Regions of the ileum, especially the terminal portion, become inflamed and oedematous, leaving normal bowel in between – 'skip lesions' – which gives it the alternative name of *regional ileitis*. The areas affected by oedema develop deep cracks which give them a cobblestone appearance, and these fissures may extend through the wall of the bowel to join with other surfaces and form *fistulae*. This extension of the inflammation leads to tangled, adherent loops of bowel known as *adhesions*, and it is these that are responsible for a lot of the colicky pain which the disease causes.

The condition starts quite suddenly in teenagers or young adults, with pain in the lower abdomen, fever and diarrhoea, so it is easily mistaken for appendicitis. There is usually an inflamed mass of tender bowel palpable in the right iliac fossa, and this may even cause an obstruction to the bowel and severe colic. The disease may resolve itself in a few weeks or run a chronic course with recurrent episodes for months or years and lead to complications. These include *malabsorption* and *anaemia, fistula formation, strictures* and *obstruction*. Because the whole body is involved symptoms outside the bowel such as clubbing of the fingers, arthritis, uveitis and ankylosing spondylitis are not uncommon.

Infections by bacteria, viruses and protozoa as well as infestations by parasites may lead to malabsorption under certain circumstances, especially if they become chronic. These are described in chapter 3 in the section on gastroenteritis.

APPENDIX

This has long been thought of as a vestigial organ with only a nuisance value when it malfunctions. However, it does contain a large amount of lymphoid tissue and may play an important part in fighting infection, a sort of 'tonsil of the intestine'. Like the tonsils it is most active between the ages of 6 and 20, and this is the age when appendicitis is most likely to occur. And like the tonsil it may inflame and even form an appendix abscess, the equivalent of a quinsy, but since it is not visible, the safest procedure has always been appendicectomy.

The first symptom of appendicitis is pain, generally colicky and in the umbilical region. The person feels nauseous and may vomit, and may sometimes get dysuria if the appendix happens to lie over the ureter, which is rather misleading. There is usually a slight fever and furred tongue with foul breath at this point, and the pain then usually localises halfway between the umbilicus and the iliac crest on the right – *McBurney's point* – which indicates that the appendix is acutely inflamed and likely to perforate. There will be tenseness of the abdominal muscles, and pain if they are pressed gently and then released, *rebound tenderness*.

Appendicitis either resolves, and this may happen many times in a so-called 'grumbling appendix', or go on to perforate, in which case an *appendix abscess* will usually form. This is allowed to settle down for several weeks and then either drained or removed. Occasionally a ruptured appendix is followed by the spread of pus throughout the peritoneal cavity and generalised *peritonitis* results.

LARGE INTESTINE

Here water is absorbed from the stools, at a rate which depends on the speed of flow of the products of digestion through the colon. Thus excessive peristaltic activity will lead to diarrhoea, and delay to constipation. The former is symptomatic of most inflammatory conditions and if these are very severe may be accompanied by the passage of fresh blood. Diarrhoea may also be caused by anxiety, malabsorption and thyrotoxicosis, as well as by local pathology.

Constipation, the infrequent passage of hard stools, is likely to occur particularly in those who consume a so-called 'low residue' diet which contains little roughage or fibre. This gives little stimulus to the bowel which becomes sluggish, and is especially a problem in the elderly whose muscles are weak. In them, and in some children who are reluctant to move their bowels, large quantities of faeces build up and impact so that finally they become incontinent. Constipation also occurs during a pyrexial illness, dehydration from any cause, obstruction by a carcinoma or any other cause, hypothyroidism and in those who avoid defaecation on account of pain from piles or an anal fissure.

COLITIS

Colitis is to the large intestine what enteritis is to the small, that is to say it refers generally to inflammatory conditions characterised by pain and diarrhoea (sometimes an infection of both is referred to as an 'entero-colitis'). There are two types of colitis, ulcerative colitis and what used to be called mucous colitis but is now more commonly known as irritable bowel or spastic colon.

Irritable bowel syndrome is a common disorder of the lower bowel whereby the regular waves of peristalsis become unco-ordinated and generate colicky pains, diarrhoea and constipation. The stools often contain an excessive amount of mucus and sometimes there is much flatulence with abdominal distension and fearful rumblings ('borborygmi'). Not uncommonly the need to hurry to the toilet arises after meals, especially breakfast, and the person is then well for the rest of the day. The pains are dull and cramplike, and may be felt anywhere in the abdomen which can be confusing, but most often in the left iliac fossa. The condition is more common in women than in men, especially those of an anxious disposition, and is seen between the ages of 20–40. What is conspicuously absent is the evidence of serious consequences such as anaemia, weight loss or bleeding, and the general health is usually good. In a given case a pattern usually develops in which there tends to be a preponderance of either diarrhoea or constipation as the main symptom.

The causes of irritable bowel are uncertain, but emotional factors often play a part, and some are overtly depressed. The illness is in many ways the female equivalent of a duodenal ulcer with its occurrence in tense, overconscientious people, often with exacerbations before a period. Food sensitivity is thought to be a factor and it may be of benefit to exclude such substances as wheat, milk and other dairy foods, tea, coffee and oranges from the diet. It is also possible that infection by Candida may initiate damage to the bowel wall and permit allergens to enter in large quantities, creating a response in the nerves of the bowel mucosa. Recently it has been shown that disturbances of the autonomic nervous system also develop in other organs at the same time, in particular the bladder, gall bladder and lungs, indicating that this is a multi-system disease.

Ulcerative colitis is altogether a more serious form of colitis

Involving especially the descending colon and rectum (the latter is termed a *proctitis*). It is relatively common among younger adults in their 20s and 30s, but the cause is unknown. One theory is that it is a result of an abnormal response by the immune system to a strain of E. coli organisms which reside in the lower bowel, for many of the patients possess autoantibodies against their own bowel mucosa. In some cases there is considerable improvement from avoiding milk and dairy products, and this should be tried. Whatever the cause, the result is a series of extensive ragged ulcers in the wall of the colon which leave areas of relatively normal but very swollen tissue in between which are known as 'pseudopolyps'.

As might be expected the main symptoms are abdominal pain and diarrhoea accompanied by bleeding and thin mucus which oozes from the ulcers, and this leads rapidly to dehydration and anaemia in a severe case. The diarrhoea characteristically continues through the night, which helps to identify its cause, and it is accompanied by a fever and rapid loss of weight during an acute attack. Most of these episodes pass within a few days or weeks, but may relapse at any time. Occasionally an ulcer becomes deep enough to perforate the wall and cause peritonitis which is extremely serious, or the bowel becomes paralysed and bowel sounds cease ('toxic dilatation'). In this case it may be necessary to operate and create a *colostomy*, which involves making an artificial anus by bringing the bowel out on to the abdominal wall and allowing the unused part to recover.

In some the disease persists as ill health and constant diarrhoea from a bowel that has partly healed but become scarred and rigid, sometimes leading to strictures. Another complication which may occur after a number of years is malignant change in the bowel wall and bowel cancer is more common in those with ulcerative colitis. Like Crohn's disease a number of systemic complications may arise in the course of time, the main ones being arthritis and skin problems.

DIVERTICULAR DISEASE

Western society has over the past century progressively refined its diet so that much of the fibre has been removed, which means that the bulk of the stools entering the colon is considerably reduced. This in turn increases the transit time and makes the stool harder to pass, requiring increased pressures of peristalsis. Over the years this takes a toll on the musculature of the colon which is then liable to give way at its weakest point, this being at the sides, where the blood vessels enter. The result is the formation of small herniations known as diverticuli. These are often present unknowingly in the elderly, a condition known as *diverticulosis*, and no great harm is done unless one of them becomes blocked and inflamed, which usually happens in the pelvic part of the colon and is then called *diverticulitis*.

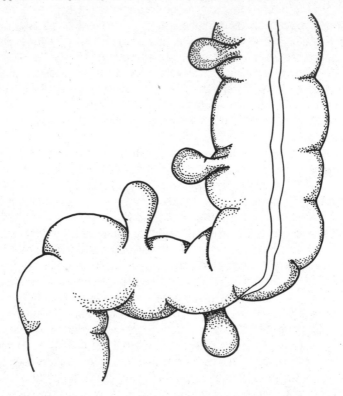

FIGURE 13.2   *Diverticuli in descending and sigmoid colon*

A condition very similar to that of appendicitis results, and indeed the symptoms are virtually identical but on the left side of the abdomen, and of course in a much older age group. Initially there is colicky pain and then later an abscess may form which will cause a fever and a tender mass in the left iliac fossa which may go on to rupture. Because the site of the abscess is at the entry of the blood vessel, heavy *rectal bleeding* may be the first sign of the disease, and there will often be either diarrhoea or constipation and sometimes even obstruction of the bowel. These symptoms are also extremely similar to those of a carcinoma of the colon, and as both conditions occur at around the same age the diagnosis is sometimes in doubt.

BOWEL CANCER

Cancer of the colon or rectum is the commonest cancer of the digestive tract in Western countries, even more frequent in appearance than stomach cancer and closely related to the standard of living. There is considerable evidence that this relates not only to the relative lack of fibre in the diet but to the large amounts of protein and to a lesser extent fat which are acted upon by the bowel bacteria to create potential carcinogens. Possibly on account of this, two thirds of the cancers occur in the terminal part of the colon – the sigmoid and the rectum, which may be just as well since they are diagnosed more early here because they are more likely to lead to an obstruction and call attention to themselves. Conditions which predispose to malignant change include longstanding *ulcerative colitis* (at one time the bowel was removed prophylactically), the presence of *polyps* in the colon and the removal of the gallbladder increases one's chances slightly.

The symptoms are either *rectal bleeding* (which is liable to be dismissed as piles), a change in bowel habit to either constipation or diarrhoea, or a dull ache in the left iliac fossa or lower abdomen. Cancer of the ascending colon seldom causes an obstruction until it has been present for some time, and as the early symptoms are vague the prognosis is correspondingly worse. Eventually spread occurs to the local lymphatics, and then to the liver causing enlargement and *jaundice*, and to the peritoneum causing *ascites*.

RECTUM & ANUS

Haemorrhoids, or *piles* as they are more commonly known, are varicose veins of the anal margin and as such have similar causes to those of the leg. Most cases occur spontaneously due to an inherited weakness of the vessel wall but some follow compression of the circulation such as that caused by pregnancy, constipation or even a tumour. The first symptom of piles is usually painless bleeding or, if they are beginning to prolapse, a mucoid discharge and some itching. Blood is noticed when the bowels are moved (haemorrhoids means 'flowing blood'), sometimes in quite large quantities, and if this continues for several months the patient may even develop iron deficiency anaemia.

The attack of piles may clear up or progress to form swellings which prolapse outside the anal margin (*second degree piles*) during defaecation but can be replaced by the patient afterwards for comfort. If they remain outside the anal margin, like the proverbial bunch of grapes, then their blood supply is likely to be cut off and they are then said to be *strangulated piles* or 'third degree haemorrhoids', which is an extremely painful

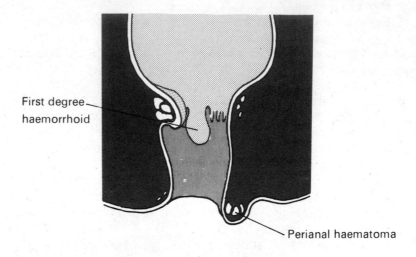

First degree haemorrhoid

Perianal haematoma

FIGURE 13.3   *A. First degree haemorrhoids in upper anal canal,*
with a perianal haematoma

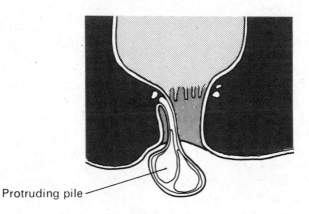

Protruding pile

FIGURE 13.3   *B. Third degree haemorrhoids*

condition. Eventually they turn a dark shade of purple and atrophy after 2–3 weeks and vanish, leaving only a small tag of skin as a reminder.

Other anal conditions are sometimes mistaken for an attack of piles, and these are:

– *Anal fissure*: a small crack, usually at the posterior margin of the anus which may appear after the passage of a hard stool, and persist for some time to cause pain and constipation.

– *Peri-anal haematoma*: a small cherry-red lump appears suddenly at the anal margin after straining, looking very like a pile but due to sudden rupture of a vein. It is painful but subsides within a few days.

– *Anal fistula*: a fistula is an abnormal communication between two mucosal surfaces, and at the anus this may occur from Crohn's disease or sometimes after an abscess at the anal margin.

– *Rectal dyschezia*: a mysterious condition characterised by sudden, severe, neuralgic pain of the rectum, anus or even genitalia and occurring spontaneously or occasionally during orgasm. It subsides after a few seconds with no ill-effects but is extremely distressing. The cause is unknown. (Gr. kezo = to ease oneself, i.e. to move one's bowels).

CHAPTER FOURTEEN

LIVER:
DISORDERS OF
MANUFACTURE &
DESTRUCTION

*T*he function of the liver, the largest gland in the body, can be likened to that of an enormous factory where raw materials enter and are converted, stored and finally despatched or broken down with the aid of innumerable enzymes. Infection or destruction of the liver will thus affect a very large number of different functions, as will blockage of the inflow or outflow tracts, and diseases of the liver reflect this by causing enlargement (*hepatomegaly*), destruction of the cells (*cirrhosis*), overflow of bile into the blood disorders or chronic infections.

HEPATOMEGALY

The liver is not normally palpable, being well hidden up under the ribs, and if it can be felt this indicates that all is not well (except in the case of young babies whose liver is working overtime to synthesize protein for growth and break down foetal blood cells, and is therefore normally palpable). The usual reasons for enlargement are *hepatitis, cirrhosis* or *tumour*, and occasionally certain blood disorders or chronic infections.

Acute viral hepatitis is the commonest liver disease and is an enormous problem worldwide, being related very largely to standards of hygiene and sanitation. Viral infections of the liver can occur with the Epstein-Barr and cytomegalovirus, as well as yellow fever, but the term 'viral hepatitis' is used to refer to that caused by a group of three viruses known as hepatitis A, B and 'non A, non B' (see below). In all three types the symptoms are very similar though there are differences in the outcome and mode of transmission.

Hepatitis A, which also goes by the name of *infectious hepatitis*, has an incubation period of about 2–6 weeks and is spread by the oral-faecal route, especially among the young, so small epidemics appear in schools and institutions from time to time. The time when the virus is being excreted the most is in the week before jaundice begins, and once this has started the individual is not infectious and specific precautions are unnecessary.

In young children the symptoms are usually extremely mild, and

In tropical countries most adults have antibodies to the virus with no previous history of the disease. Where there are symptoms, these come on over a few days as a fever with marked *anorexia, nausea, diarrhoea* and upper *abdominal discomfort*, the liver being enlarged and tender. Soon a faint tinge of *jaundice* will usually, but not always, appear and the stools go pale, but this seldom lasts more than a week or two, although the itching of the skin which sometimes accompanies it may linger and full recovery take many months. Damage to the liver is rarely severe but alcohol should be avoided for a year. On very rare occasions there is severe illness and death from acute liver failure.

Hepatitis B or *serum hepatitis* is spread by direct contact with the blood, saliva or semen of an infected person or a carrier, hence its occurrence in intravenous drug addicts, homosexual or bisexual men (for reasons similar to AIDS – see chapter 2), recipients of blood transfusions and sometimes dentists and those working in dialysis units. It is also considerably more likely to occur in immigrants from Africa, Asia or the Mediterranean, and in those who live in institutions for the mentally handicapped.

The incubation period is longer, 2–6 months, and the disease is seen mostly in young men as opposed to schoolchildren. The onset is slower and often accompanied by a rash, but the symptoms more severe than type A. There is often arthritis and a considerable degree of jaundice, and the infection may persist for a long time, some patients even remaining carriers of the virus long after they have recovered. In order to confirm the diagnosis the blood is examined for evidence of the viral antigen, known as 'Australia antigen' because it was first discovered in the blood of an aborigine. The immediate outlook for hepatitis B is good, although a small number develop chronic hepatitis. In the long term, however, the disruption of the liver cells means that there is a high incidence of eventual cirrhosis or liver cancer.

Hepatitis non A non B is a somewhat clumsy title which merely indicates that as yet the agent(s) are unknown. It is a waterborne disease found especially in India with a degree of severity somewhere between the other two.

CIRRHOSIS

The word comes from the Greek meaning 'tawny', and refers to the greyish-brown discoloration which the liver undergoes when its cells are injured and the original architecture of the delicate lobules is replaced by a scarred battleground of fibrous tissue. Cirrhosis is classically associated with longstanding *alcoholism*, but may also appear after *hepatitis* or as a result of *heart failure*. A particular type of cirrhosis, occurring mostly in women, arises as a result of sluggishness in the flow of bile due to an autoimmune connective tissue disorder, and is called *primary biliary cirrhosis*.

Most of these causes start by inflaming the liver and making it swell in a variety of different ways, and each has a specific pathological characteristic when seen under a microscope. So the liver may start as a swollen 'fatty liver', but then gradually shrinks as fibrosis overtakes the attempts at regeneration and finally ends up as a shrivelled 'nodular liver'. Naturally, many functions of the liver are affected which in the extreme case may fail altogether – *liver failure* or 'hepatocellular failure' – and this is the endpoint of several different kinds of liver disorders. There are simply not enough cells left to carry out the functions of the organ, and a number of clinical features ensue:

- wasting, due to the inability to form proteins.
- ascites (Gr. askos = a wineskin) due to the low plasma proteins (the presence of proteins in the plasma normally draws fluid out of the tissues by osmosis).
- spider naevi, due to dilation of the capillaries in the skin of the face and neck.
- gynaecomastia (male breast enlargement), due to inability to break down sex hormones, particularly oestrogens.
- testicular atrophy and impotence for the same reasons.
- jaundice, due to failure of bilirubin metabolism.
- portal hypertension (see below).
- eventually coma and death from the build up of toxic waste especially ammonia.

PORTAL HYPERTENSION

You will recall that the liver has blood delivered to it by both the hepatic artery, supplying oxygen, and the portal vein, supplying the products of digestion directly from that part of the digestive tract lying within the peritoneum. If the branches of the portal vein become blocked, as may happen either through a tumour or cirrhosis, the back-pressure will start to cause oedema and engorgement of the gut, much in the way that left ventricular failure engorges the lungs. This means that the abdominal organs will swell up considerably, especially the spleen to cause enlargement of that organ (*splenomegaly*), and the blood will be forced into alternative routes.

There are three of these alternatives – the oesophageal vein at the top of the system, the haemorrhoidal vein at the bottom and the long defunct umbilical vein at the centre. All these have potential connections with the rest of the venous circulation and can be used to re-route the blood back to the heart. This means that the patient with portal hypertension will start to develop *piles* and swollen *oesophageal varices*, distended varicose veins in the lower oesophagus near the cardiac sphincter, the rupture of which is followed by a torrential haemorrhage and haematemesis. If the umbilical vein is called into use then a delta of distended veins may be seen radiating from the umbilicus – the so-called Medusa's head or 'caput Medusae'.

JAUNDICE

In this state the small amount of bile which we normally have circulating in our blood is increased to the point where it becomes visible first in the sclera and then in the skin. This increase may be due to one of three reasons (see figure 14.1):

– the red cells are being broken down in numbers too great for the liver to cope. This is *haemolytic* or *pre-hepatic jaundice*.

– the liver cells are damaged and cannot conjugate the bile salts, *hepatocellular jaundice*.

– there is a blockage in the bile duct preventing outflow, *obstructive* or *post-hepatic jaundice*.

Haemolytic jaundice is uncommon except in certain blood disorders such as sickle-cell anaemia, thalassaemia, pernicious anaemia and rhesus disease, or in malaria. The jaundice is seldom very severe as the liver can cope with most of the bilirubin, but the simultaneous presence of anaemia gives these patients a characteristic lemon-yellow tinge.

Hepatocellular jaundice has already been mentioned in association with viral hepatitis, and there are many other agents which will damage the liver cells, particularly alcohol and drugs such as paracetamol, largactil and some antidepressants, as well as poisons such as phosphorus and the amanita fungi. These often have the effect of swelling the tissues which obstruct the outflow of whatever bile is formed, a situation called 'biliary stasis'. A similar situation arises in the familiar *neonatal jaundice*, when the immature liver is unable to conjugate the large amount of bilirubin because its enzymes have not yet fully formed. This process of conjugation is therefore sometimes aided by stimulating similar enzymes in the skin by using UV light, in order to prevent a build-up of bilirubin. If this exceeds a certain level in the blood, it tends to deposit in the brain and cause a form of damage termed *kernicterus* ('icterus' means jaundiced and Kera was the goddess of destruction).

Obstructive jaundice arises as a result either of compression of the bile duct by a tumour, or from a gallstone. As no bile flows, there is an increasingly deepening level of jaundice with pale, clay-coloured stools and dark urine. The circulating bile leads to itching of the skin and a metallic taste in the mouth, and if a stone is present there will usually be colicky pain.

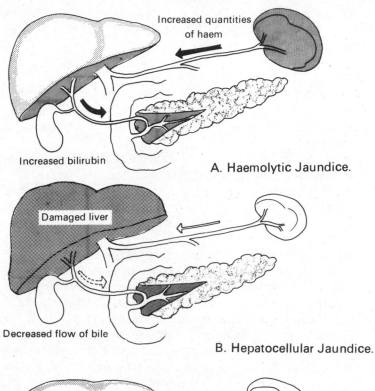

Increased quantities of haem

Increased bilirubin

A. Haemolytic Jaundice.

Damaged liver

Decreased flow of bile

B. Hepatocellular Jaundice.

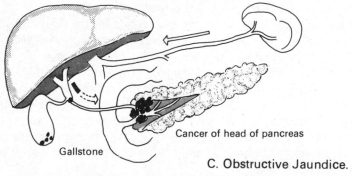

Cancer of head of pancreas

Gallstone

C. Obstructive Jaundice.

FIGURE 14.1   *The different causes of jaundice*

Tumours arising in the liver are known as *hepatomas*, and are rare in this country but the commonest cancer on a worldwide basis. Most Western cancers obstructing bile outflow are found to arise in the head of the pancreas, or more commonly as secondary tumours which have metastasised from the colon or stomach, and which swell the lymphatics at the exit of the bile duct from the liver.

Gallstones are discussed in detail in the next section.

GALLSTONES

This common condition increases in frequency with age, but does so more rapidly in women so that young women are more likely to suffer from *cholelithiasis*, as stones are sometimes called, than young men but the incidence evens up later on. Oestrogens appear to be a factor as gallstones are associated with having children, diabetes and taking the contraceptive pill, and there is still a modicum of truth in the adage about the 'fair, fat, fertile and flatulent'. A highly refined carbohydrate diet is another factor, as the synthesis of cholesterol in the bile is increased, but the question of what exactly causes gallstones has no simple answer, and there is more than a single cause as although the majority of stones contain cholesterol a few consist only of bile pigments.

Because the chief function of the gallbladder is to concentrate bile by a factor of about twelve times, there is always a risk that cholesterol, the main bile salt, will crystallise and form a nucleus around which other substances can deposit. The majority of those with stones in the gallbladder do not know it as they have no symptoms. Some get a vague feeling of discomfort and flatulence, particularly after a fatty meal, called 'flatulent dyspepsia', but this may happen for other reasons also, such as hiatus hernia. An unfortunate minority suffer from more severe consequences such as biliary colic or cholecystitis.

Biliary colic is the name given to the pain which accompanies the passage of a stone down the bile duct. This may happen when the gallbladder contracts after a meal, causing a sudden pain in the epigastrium which becomes steadily worse with sweating, vomiting and extreme restlessness. It is felt mainly in the upper abdomen but may also radiate to the lower end of the right scapula or the shoulder tip, and continues steadily for some hours, ceasing only when the stone has passed into the duodenum. If the stone takes more than a few hours to pass then the resulting obstruction to bile leads to a degree of jaundice with pale stools and darkening of the urine.

In some the stone becomes impacted in the neck of the gallbladder and leads to pain after meals when the gland contracts, and also to

TABLE 14.1	Possible causes of abdominal pain (N.B. Site may vary)

Condition	Pointers
Upper abdomen	
Hiatus hernia	Epigastric, dyspepsia, heartburn, hiccough
Gastric ulcer	Pain after food, vomiting, relief from milk
Duodenal ulcer	Pain before food, periodicity, nocturnal
Cholecystitis	Site, fever, flatulence, referred shoulder
Gallstones	Colicky pain, flatulence, possibly jaundice
Pneumonia	Cough, fever, chest signs
Myocardial infarct	Sudden onset, sweating, pallor, nausea
Pancreatitis	Shock, fever, guarding
Pancreatic tumour	Chronic pain to back, worse lying, jaundice
Lower abdomen	
Dysmenorrhoea	Regular, related to periods, colicky
Cystitis	Dysuria, blood in urine, frequency
Irritable bowel syn	Regular pattern, constipation/diarrhoea
Endometriosis	Backache before periods, painful intercourse
Pelvic inf disease	Discharge, urethritis, fever, perhaps a coil
Prostatitis	Pain in perineum, dysuria, urethral discharge
Lateral pain (left or right)	
Appendicitis	McBurney's point, rebound, furred tongue
Pyelonephritis	Rigors, loin tenderness, cloudy urine
Ovulation pain	Timing, brevity
Renal colic	Pain worse on jolting, radiation, haematuria
Ectopic pregnancy	Abrupt onset, missed period, bleeding
Diverticulitis	Colicky pain, constipation, age, haemorrhage
Central pain (variable)	
Early appendicitis	Colicky pain, furred tongue, fever, diarrhoea
Gastroenteritis	Colicky pain, furred tongue, fever, diarrhoea
Food allergy	Regularly after certain foods, allergic type
Mesenteric adenitis	Child, upper respiratory infection, glands
Crohn's disease	Colicky pain, weight loss, fever, anaemia
Abdominal aneurysm	Abrupt severe pain radiating to back, shock

stagnation of the bile which cannot escape. This state of affairs will eventually end with the bile becoming infected, causing an acute inflammation or *cholecystitis*. There is a fever, malaise and tenderness over the liver, sometimes with a tinge of jaundice if the duct is also inflamed. This may be a recurrent situation every time the patient consumes fatty food, and eventually the gallbladder will become shrivelled, functionless and liable to malignancy, and is therefore often removed by the operation of 'cholecystectomy'.

CHAPTER FIFTEEN

KIDNEYS: DISORDERS OF EXCRETION

*T*he predominant function of the kidney is to maintain a constant internal water and mineral balance, and to eliminate waste and surplus material. Its huge powers of filtration and secretion allow the kidney to monitor the volume, acidity, toxicity and mineral content of the whole circulation every 30 minutes or so, for one fifth of the output from the heart travels down the renal arteries. This means that the function of the renal tubules is vital, and although we possess a large reserve and can even manage on a single kidney, diseases of the substance or *parenchyma* of the kidney may damage the delicate filtration in one of three main ways. These are, very broadly speaking, through inflammation of the filter (*nephritis*), by perforation of the filter with 'holes' (*nephrosis*), and by total blockage of the filter (*renal failure*).

As well as this constant adjustment of the blood, two other important functions related to this are performed by the kidney. These are the control of blood pressure by the hormone renin which the glomerular cells secrete, and the stimulation of erythrocyte production by the secretion of erythropoietin in response to anoxia, and both these mechanisms may go awry and lead to hypertension, anaemia or even polycythaemia.

A variety of terms are used in describing renal disease, the main ones being as follows:
- *Anuria*: absence of urinary output from the kidney.
- *Retention*: inability to pass urine present in the bladder.
- *Oliguria*: passage of scanty urine from the kidney.
- *Polyuria*: passage of large quantities of urine ('diuresis').
- *Haematuria*: passing blood in the urine.
- *Glycosuria*: passing glucose in the urine.
- *Proteinuria*: passing protein in the urine (=albuminuria).
- *Dysuria*: painful passage of urine.
- *Incontinence*: involuntary passage of urine.
- *Micturition*: the act of urination.
- *Strangury*: constant urge to urinate but with the painful passage of only one or two drops of (bloodstained) urine.

ACUTE GLOMERULONEPHRITIS (NEPHRITIS)

In 1827 Richard Bright gave a classic description of a disease he called 'acute nephritis', and which has since come to be known as Bright's disease or acute glomerulonephritis (AGN). He noticed that some people, usually children, develop a feverish illness with a puffy face and pain in the loins about 2 weeks after a sore throat or attack of tonsillitis. The urine is scanty (oliguria) and either bloodstained or discoloured and smoky, depending on the amount of haematuria. Because excessive salt and water is retained in the body the blood pressure is raised and the child develops swollen legs and eyelids. Most of these children recover fully within a week or so, and this recovery is announced by a diuresis with a marked polyuria, but a few have a prolonged period of anuria, sometimes lasting 4–6 weeks.

From subsequent investigations it seems that certain strains of streptococci and occasionally other organisms provoke an antibody reaction by the immune system, and that these antibodies go on to damage the cells lining Bowman's capsule, which have a similar antigenic structure, resulting in their inflammation. Since Bright's time the advent of the electron microscope has enabled the distinction of many different types of changes in the glomeruli to be made, and this has lead to a complex classification of nephritis, such as 'proliferative', 'membranous' etc, but all have the hallmarks of *haematuria, proteinuria, oedema* and *oliguria.*

One particular variety of glomerulonephritis which is due to an allergic reaction to an unknown agent is 'Henoch-Schonlein purpura'. It is seen in children after an acute fever, and they develop a tendency to bleed from the capillaries. The symptoms are therefore a purpuric (haemorrhagic) rash on the legs and buttocks, with pains and swellings in the joints, abdominal colic and even bleeding from the bowel in addition to the nephritis with haematuria.

RENAL FAILURE

When the kidneys fail they are no longer able to secrete urine, and so the three main constituents of the blood – water, salt and urea – build up in the body causing *oedema, hypertension and uraemia.* Urea is extremely toxic to the body when present in excessive amounts and before the advent of dialysis the patient was usually in a uraemic coma by the end of a week or so, and died within a fortnight (much more rapidly than was the case with nephritis where the kidneys held out for weeks even in a severe case).

Acute renal failure occurs suddenly if the blood supply is abruptly shut off and this may happen after a heart attack, massive haemorrhage, overwhelming infection or severe dehydration. This results in the death of large numbers of kidney tubules ('tubular necrosis'), which do not have the power of recovery, and in temporary damage to many more. A similar result occurs when the tubules are poisoned by certain drugs, particularly some antibiotics like streptomycin, or after severe burns or crush injuries where large amounts of tissue are destroyed. There is then complete *anuria* and in order to slow down the rate of accumulation of urea it is important that the patient restricts the amount of protein consumed to a bare minimum, and also the amount of fluid drunk so they do not become 'waterlogged'. The symptoms of anorexia, nausea, vomiting, headache and hiccough increase unless the level of urea in the blood is lowered either spontaneously or by dialysis.

Damage to the kidney by diabetes mellitus, hypertension, infection (pyelonephritis), polycystic disease and sometimes renal stones, may lead to failure of the kidneys of a rather more leisurely sort, **chronic renal failure**. Here sufficient urine is passed but the concentrating power of the kidney is lost, so it is very dilute and tends to occur at night (*nocturia*). Because the production of erythropoietin is damaged there is almost always a degree of anaemia present too, and this condition runs a steady downhill course so it is these patients who are most likely to be offered renal transplants.

NEPHROTIC SYNDROME (NEPHROSIS)

Some cases of nephritis never really recover and the glomeruli, despite patching themselves up after the inflammation, remain 'leaky'. This means that the larger molecules in the plasma will start to escape, especially the plasma proteins – the smaller globulins at first and then even the larger albumen. So the hallmark of nephrotic syndrome is *proteinuria*, and very large amounts of albumen and globulins may be lost to the body which make the urine cloudy causing it to froth up in the toilet bowl. More seriously, the liver cannot synthesize albumen fast enough to keep pace with the loss, even though the patient is on a high protein diet, and so the plasma protein level begins to drop.

This has two major consequences. Firstly the patient becomes very oedematous, often with *ascites*, because the plasma proteins are of major importance in maintaining the osmotic pressure of the blood. If they are not present in sufficient numbers then there is no suction force from the blood to draw the water back into the capillaries from inside the body tissues (you will recollect from physiology that sugars break down into water and CO_2). This leaves all the cells waterlogged and gives the person the classic puffy appearance. Secondly they lack sufficient immunoglobulins to withstand infections which are therefore frequent. The typical clinical picture is a pale, anaemic individual who is swollen and oedematous but whose muscles are actually wasted because they lack protein, and who tends to suffer from repeated infectious illness. Not all cases of nephrotic syndrome are a result of glomerulonephritis, for sometimes diabetes mellitus and systemic lupus (SLE) may cause it, as may treatment with gold injections for rheumatoid arthritis.

RENAL STONES AND OBSTRUCTION

Stones or calculi are formed from crystals of substances present in urine which precipitate either because the urine is very concentrated, as occurs in chronic unaccustomed dehydration (the troops in North Africa during the last war frequently developed renal calculi) or because abnormal substances are present. These take the form of *calcium* salts which are excreted in large quantities when the patient is immobilised or drinks large amounts of milk, *uric acid* stones which may form in gout and *phosphate* stones in the presence of renal infection. It must be said, however, that in most cases of renal stones no abnormal constituents of the diet or urine can be found, though stones are known to be rare in vegetarians.

Most renal stones form in the pelvis or calcyces of the kidney, and enlarge slowly to cause a dull pain in the loin which is worse when the patient is jarred. The stone may on occasions reach a very large size, occupying the whole of the renal pelvis and branching into the calyces – a *staghorn calculus*. More commonly it will pass down the ureter when it is the size of a grape seed, producing as it does the agony of *renal colic*. This is a sharp, severe pain which is referred from the loin down into the groin and testis (stones are much more common in men) and causes much restlessness in the patient as well as nausea, vomiting and sweating as he rolls about the bed. The pain is continuous and periodically increases in severity as the stone is squeezed a little further down the ureter, until it is eventually released into the bladder, from where there is little trouble passing it. The urine will be scanty and bloodstained, and sometimes infection will set in if the obstruction has been present for more than a few days.

At one time bladder stones were common in this country, and created chronic cystitis and severe strangury, as those familiar with the writings of Samuel Johnson will know. They appear to be a consequence of longstanding infection which may have been produced by the urethral strictures which follow untreated gonorrhoea, as well as to dietary factors which may explain the frequency of bladder stones in parts of Asia still.

Obstruction to the outflow of urine from the kidney not only leads to infection but may, if chronic, cause the pelvis and calyces to dilate and exert back-pressure on the tubules so that filtration can no longer occur. This situation is called a *hydronephrosis* and eventually the kidney becomes a cyst containing urine with little kidney substance left. The enlarged kidney may be palpable and there is often sediment in the urine and aching after drinking a lot of fluid, but the diagnosis is established by performing an intravenous pyelogram (IVP). This is the standard method of examining the kidney and ureters by injecting a radio-opaque dye into a vein which the kidney picks up and rapidly excretes, outlining the urinary tract on X-ray as it does so and also giving a measure of its function. Stones will show up as small gaps in the dye as it flows down the ureter.

Polycystic disease is a similar condition affecting not only the kidneys but sometimes also the liver and pancreas as well. It is a congenital condition and when the kidneys are affected there are multiple cysts throughout its substance, some of which may be very large. The outcome depends on the amount of renal tissue which is damaged by pressure from the cysts, and whether renal failure, hypertension or infection supervene, any of which may shorten the life of the individual concerned.

URINARY INFECTIONS

Under normal circumstances the urinary trace is sterile. When infections occur these usually enter via the urethra from below and travel upwards, especially in the case of women as the urethra is short, straight and relatively wide. The invading organism is usually the commensal bacterium present in the gut, E. coli, which is also found on the skin of the perineum. It may sometimes exist in the bladder without causing symptoms, a situation called 'bacteriuria' and often occurring in pregnancy, because of the high level of circulating oestrogens which tends to dilate the urinary passages.

More often, however, there is a sense of discomfort and frequency of micturition accompanied by dysuria and even strangury, which is typical of *cystitis*. This is a common condition, especially in pregnancy for the reasons above, and some women suffer from multiple episodes. In many of these there is no evidence of infection when a mid-stream specimen of urine is cultured, and the name *irritable bladder* or *trigonitis* is used instead. This may result from trauma or allergy, and be worse after intercourse and if nylon tights or vaginal deodorants are used. Any condition causing stagnation of the flow of urine predisposes to infection, and it is thus commonly seen in pregnancy, prostatism and where stones are present, when the infection is likely to ascend further and involve the kidney itself, causing pyelonephritis.

Acute pyelonephritis, sometimes called *pyelitis*, is an infection of the pelvis and deeper renal tissues and may occur without a previous cystitis, as happens quite often in pregnancy. The first symptoms are a sudden high *fever* with *rigors* (uncontrollable shivering), *aching in the loins* and usually nausea and *vomiting*. Both kidneys are generally involved and there is scanty, bloodstained urine containing pus cells. Some cases occur in children who develop recurrent attacks early in life because they have a congenital abnormality in the valves of the bladder so the urine flows back up into the kidney as the bladder contracts during micturition, causing dilation and stagnation – *ureteric reflux*.

If the infection is not successfully eradicated then it may slowly penetrate into the parenchyma of the kidney and cause patchy areas of fibrosis and scarring of the nephrons so that over the years the kidneys shrink in size and *chronic pyelonephritis* results. There are usually few if any symptoms apart from general ill-health but eventually the renal function is compromised and hypertension develops.

Renal tuberculosis is an exception to the general rule of infection ascending from below, and is usually carried to the kidney from a focus in the lungs or the gut by way of the blood stream. There it causes the typical caseation which breaks through a calyx and tubercle bacilli leak into the urine to cause inflammation of the bladder and epididymis. There are few specific signs, however, and unless the urine is examined for blood and pus cells the condition, though uncommon, can be overlooked.

TUMOURS

The urinary tract is a place through which many chemicals, some of them potential carcinogens, are passed in high concentration, and it is therefore not surprising when either the kidney nephron or, more frequently, the lining of the bladder, undergoes neoplastic change.

Renal carcinomas arise in the delicate cells of the walls of the tubules and gradually compress the surrounding tissues before breaking out directly through the capsule of the kidney or spreading via the blood to a distant organ, often the lungs or bones. The earliest symptom is almost always *haematuria* which gives a grey tinge to the urine unless it is profuse, but sometimes a dragging pain in the loin develops or even a sudden renal colic from a clot of blood. The bleeding is characteristically of an intermittent nature and usually occurs in the older age group. Renal cancer is also notorious for causing a protracted malaise and intermittent fever for many weeks before it is discovered and should always be considered as a possibility in these circumstances.

The transitional cells which line the ureters and bladder are much more likely to develop malignant change than their renal counterparts, especially in those who smoke or consume large amounts of coffee. They arise as multiple warty growths called *papillomas*, usually in middle-aged

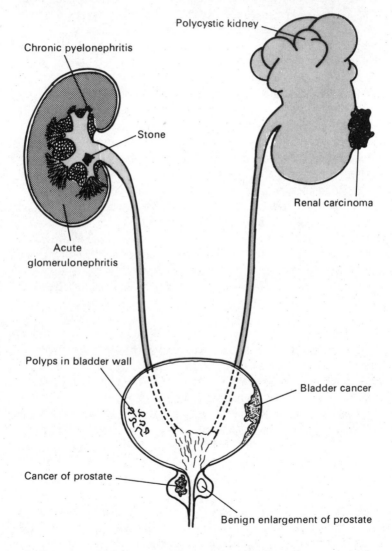

FIGURE 15.1   *Causes of haematuria*

men, and during the early stages the epithelium is unstable but not as yet cancerous. However, it is highly likely that one or more of these papillomas will eventually become invasive and infiltrate the wall of the bladder and surrounding tissues. Again, the first symptom is painless haematuria, sometimes with frequency. Later the tumour may obstruct the ureteric orifices and cause hydronephrosis of one of the kidneys. The conventional treatment of these papillomas is to remove them with a laser every few months as they occur.

THE PROSTATE GLAND

This gland, the size and shape of a chestnut, completely encircles the male urethra where it leaves the bladder and is thus intimately connected with the workings of the internal urethral sphincter. As part of the ageing process, it starts to enlarge during middle-life, and thereafter tends to become more rigid in consistency, so the combination of these two features is responsible for the symptoms of **prostatism** or *benign hypertrophy* as it is sometimes known.

The first of these is usually an increasing sluggishness of the stream of urine during urination as the urethra becomes narrowed, and also hesitancy in starting and some dribbling at the end as the sphincter fails to close completely. Because the gland is often congested with blood, a small vessel may rupture and cause a few drops of blood to be passed at the very beginning or end of micturition. As the gland enlarges, so the muscular wall of the bladder must thicken to increase the pressure necessary to void urine, but part of the gland will sometimes bulge upwards into the bladder and create a valve which can block the exit of urine suddenly and

TABLE 15.1	Possible causes of blood in the urine
Condition	**Pointers**
Cystitis	Pain on passing urine, frequency
Exercise induced	Recurrent episodes in young person
Prostatitis	Urethritis, discharge
Nephritis	Fever, puffy face, aching loins, sore throat
Calculus	Renal colic, renal ache, restlessness
Prostatic enlargement	Frequency, poor stream, dribbling, age
Pyelonephritis	Fever, rigors, loin pain, possible pregnancy
Bladder polyp	Age and sex, painless
Neoplasm	Age, painless, intermittent
Drugs	Anticoagulants
Polycystic kidneys	Aching loin, hypertension, dragging sensation

dramatically. This *acute retention* is painful and embarrassing and must be relieved by passing a catheter, but may well recur.

There is also the possibility of the high bladder pressure squeezing stagnant urine back up into the kidney and causing infection and eventual kidney failure if the prostatic problem is ignored for too long, and this is occasionally a cause of an elderly man's confusion. If this is thought to be a risk then an operation may be suggested to resect the part of the prostate which is obstructing the urethra, a 'transurethral resection' (TUR), rather than removing the whole gland as was once done.

Cancer of the prostate may well present with symptoms which are identical to those of benign hypertrophy, and a biopsy may be required to distinguish with any certainty between the two. Fortunately this form of cancer, although extremely common in old age, is so slow to progress that most of those who have it succumb eventually to something else. It is estimated that about 15% of men in their forties actually have it but only 1 in 1000 dies of the disease, and that because of secondary spread to the bones. These are usually the bones of the lower spine, or sometimes a long bone, and may result in deep bone pains so low back pains in an old man should always be regarded with some suspicion.

Prostatitis, on the other hand, is an inflammatory condition of younger men, which is sometimes a byproduct of urethritis. It usually starts suddenly, with a fever and acute pain in the perineum, the scrotum and sometimes the lower back. There is a constant desire to urinate and pain on passing urine, which is cloudy and contains mucus and pus cells. Many cases of prostatitis are related to chlamydial infections, which are partially susceptible to antibiotics, particularly tetracyclene, but sometimes no organisms can be found in the urine and the condition becomes chronic and flares up periodically at times of stress and sexual activity.

DIURETICS

These are a group of drugs used to promote a *diuresis* or increased flow of urine, thus removing excess fluid from the body. However, if the kidney is forced to pass more urine than usual, it cannot pass water alone and will of necessity include certain minerals, more correctly known as *electrolytes*, in the flow and these will also be lost. The chief one of these is potassium, which is very important for the functioning of the cells of the muscles and the heart, and without it the muscles become weak and the heart beats irregularly. Sodium, in the form of salt, is equally important for the body, but because our kidneys evolved over millions of years on the plains of Africa where salt was in short supply, the kidney developed the habit of hanging on to sodium at all costs, and always preferred to allow potassium to be discarded first. This situation is now to our disadvantage, as salt is added in abundance to so many foods and the body cannot get rid of it easily, so it remains in the tissues and blood.

The accumulation of salt means also the accumulation of water since the proportions must be the same, so we put on weight with the oedema, the volume of our blood increases and so in a roundabout way up goes the blood pressure. One solution might be to take a diuretic to get rid of the fluid and, gradually, the salt, but this would also mean replacing the potassium which is simultaneously being lost or we would enter a state of hypokalaemia (L. kalium = potassium). More sensible would be to reduce the amount of salt we eat, not an easy task as it is included in the majority of foods that we buy, mainly to make them more appetising. If the oedema is purely local, then it is pointless to take diuretics as the body will simply redistribute the remaining excess, so taking diuretics for swollen ankles makes little sense.

The two pathological reasons for general fluid retention are either because the blood has insufficient albumen (for a more complete explanation see the section on nephrotic syndrome), or because the heart is failing to pump adequately. In the latter case it may be vital to take a diuretic to survive, or the lungs will quickly fill with fluid in the form of pulmonary oedema. Hence diuretics are either needed to act suddenly and dramatically, or on a long-term slow basis.

Some of the most powerful diuretics work by preventing the kidney from reabsorbing fluid in the loop of Henle, so the bulk of it is passed out. As over 90% of the filtered urine is normally reabsorbed here, this is quickly lost, and the effect of giving a so-called 'loop diuretic' such as frusemide (Lasix) is similar to wringing out a sponge. Another way of causing a diuresis is to prevent the hormone ADH (antidiuretic hormone) from carrying out its duty on the distal tubule. You will, I hope, recall that ADH carries out the final modification on the concentration of urine passed but has no effect on the absorption of potassium, so if an 'ADH antagonist' such as spironolactone (Aldactone) is used, no potassium needs to be replaced and the action is more gentle.

The most frequently used diuretics, though, are those which act at the distal tubule but not by blocking ADH activity. These are the thiazide group of which the best-known names are bendrofluazide, Moduretic and Navidrex-K (the K in the latter indicates the addition of potassium). They are gentle in action, but usually given first thing in the morning as they act over several hours. The main unwanted effects stem from the loss of potassium incurred, as replacement is not always reliable and giving too much is equally undesirable. Occasionally giving a diuretic will increase the concentration of uric acid in the body sufficiently to provoke an acute attack of gout. Discontinuing diuretics will simply lead to a worsening of the oedema but is not generally harmful unless the person is in heart failure when they may develop an attack of pulmonary oedema.

CHAPTER SIXTEEN

HORMONES:
DISORDERS OF
CONTROL

*T*he function of the hormones is to maintain long term stabilization of the body's processes such as growth, metabolism and sex, the more immediate adjustments being left to the nervous system, although there are intimate connections between the two in the pituitary gland, the 'hypothalamo-pituitary axis'. This means that disorders of the endocrine system are generally insidious in onset but have subtle and far-reaching affects on most of the organs of the body. Although each pituitary hormone acts on a single tissue or organ, sometimes called a 'target organ', the hormones produced in turn by these target organs have a wide variety of activities which depend on a steady supply of the stimulating hormone, and most forms of pathology are therefore caused by an under or overproduction by these glands. The exception to this is diabetes mellitus, which is the commonest of all the hormonal disorders.

PITUITARY GLAND

This, the conductor of the whole glandular orchestra, is safely tucked away at the base of the brain, being accessible to the surgeon only via the upper recesses of the nose (L.pituita = catarrh). It is responsible for the production of nine hormones, despite being only the size of a peanut, and damage to the gland therefore has very far-reaching consequences. Fortunately disorders are rare, although occasionally a benign tumour will cause oversecretion, or infarction of the gland result in hypopituitarism.

Hypopituitarism, sometimes called 'Simmond's disease', is a loss of the secretions of the anterior pituitary usually as a result of a head injury or severe haemorrhage following labour (when the gland is most susceptible as it is at the greatest time of stimulation). The effect of this is the loss of hormones stimulating growth, sexual development, pigmentation and the thyroid and adrenal glands. In addition prolactin loss causes the milk to dry up in lactating mothers, and this may be the first sign. If the condition occurs before puberty the subject never grows up and remains, like Peter Pan, short and sexually underdeveloped.

Diabetes insipidus is another possible consequence of injury to the pituitary, but in this case it is the posterior lobe which is affected, resulting in a loss of antidiuretic hormone (ADH). This normally enables the kidney to conserve water by concentrating urine, so its absence results in the passage of large quantities of very dilute urine, up to four gallons a day. The main symptoms are thirst, nocturia and constipation, and the treatment usually involves taking synthetic ADH in the form of nasal drops.

Acromegaly is an example of overproduction of a pituitary hormone caused by a benign tumor (adenoma) in an adult. The hormone in question is growth hormone, and leads to enlargement of the hands, feet and jaw (Gr.acros = extremity), as well as the soft tissues. This results in a general coarsening of the features, a thick tongue, fatigue, aches and pains and increased sweating. Moreover the expanding tumour may give rise to headaches, and pressure on the nearby optic nerve lead to defects in the visual field. In the very rare event of the condition occurring in children it is known as giantism and the child or adolescent will start to develop exceptional stature if they are still in the growing phase. It is said that Goliath had just such a problem, and it was only his visual defect which enabled David to creep up on the blind side!

THYROID GLAND
Of all the glands under the influence of the pituitary, this is the one with the highest failure rate. When this happens the gland will often enlarge to form either a smooth (diffuse) or lumpy (nodular) swelling called a goitre. However, not all goitres are pathological and sometimes a so-called 'physiological goitre' is seen in normal pregnancy and in some adolescents. Goitres may occasionally be the consequence of a lack of iodine in the diet, or the consumption of excessive quantities of cabbage and similar vegetables which interfere with its uptake and are therefore termed 'goitrogens'. The thyroid is for some reason very susceptible to attack by antibodies, even those made erroneously by the body against itself (autoimmune disease), which may lead it to over- or under-producing thyroxine and cause hyperthyroidism or hypothyroidism.

Hyperthyroidism or thyrotoxicosis occurs when the thyroid escapes control of the TSH from the pituitary and begins to produce increasing quantities of thyroxine under the influence of another hormone called 'long-acting thyroid stimulator' or LATS, which acts as a sort of 'counterfeit' TSH, while TSH itself is suppressed. LATS also causes enlargement of the pad of fat behind the eye, and hence the familiar bulging eyes or exophthalmos which is a noticeable feature of what is sometimes called Grave's disease.

It is most frequently seen in young women, who notice increasing exhaustion, nervousness, insomnia, sweating and palpitations, symptoms which might easily be put down to anxiety. The increasing amount of energy being metabolised is obtained by an enlarged appetite but with a paradoxical loss of weight, while tremor of the hands is caused by the bounding circulation which also leads to high blood pressure and even atrial fibrillation and dyspnoea. Peristalsis also increases and causes diarrhoea or more frequent normal stools, while the periods become scanty or cease altogether. The eyes feel inflamed and gritty, and double vision may occur if the muscles are affected.

Such a florid picture is seldom seen, and in older people the signs may be restricted to palpitations or atrial fibrillation and wasting of the muscles, with no goitre or exophthalmos. In them it is often a small overactive *thyroid nodule* which is the problem, and this is another form of hyperthyroidism.

There are three conventional avenues of treatment – by antithyroid drugs, by removal of part of the gland (thyroidectomy) or by destruction of the gland with radioactive iodine. The drug treatment is normally tried first, but may result in relapse when the drug is stopped; surgery is the usual approach and works in the great majority but occasionally causes hypothyroidism which requires replacement with thyroxine, or a further relapse, when radioactive iodine may be recommended. This latter treatment is only reserved for the elderly, as there is a small risk of thyroid cancer or leukaemia occurring several years later.

Hypothyroidism or *myxoedema* (Gr.myxos=mucus) can be a result of pituitary failure but is much more often due to damage to the thyroid itself by inflammation, drugs such as lithium, removal of too much of the gland for thyrotoxicosis or most often from an autoimmune process causing destruction of the gland, known as *Hashimoto's disease*. The term 'myxoedema' refers to the mucilaginous substance deposited under the skin giving it a puffy, yellow, coarse appearance, but differing from true oedema in that it does not pit under pressure. It is one of the commonest and most subtle of the endocrine disorders, arising usually in middle-aged women around the time of the menopause, and leading to weakness and fatigue, rheumatic pains and loss of appetite but not weight, which may actually increase.

All bodily functions slow down, so there is mental apathy and poor memory, intellectual deterioration and a gradual impairment of efficiency which is all too often put down to ageing. Because of the effect on the nervous system, the heart rate slows down and the reflexes of the body operate slowly, so that testing the knee jerk is a useful indicator of the presence of the condition. The presence of anaemia along with an increased incidence of atheroma may well lead to angina. There is sensitivity to the cold and increasing constipation, with heavy periods and loss of interest in sex. The hair thins and becomes lifeless, the voice deepens owing to deposits of myxoedema on the vocal chords, and there may be some deafness. Myxoedema compressing the median nerve in the wrist may lead to carpal tunnel syndrome with tingling of the fingers and a tendency to drop things. Eventually, if not diagnosed and treated the condition terminates in coma preceded by paranoid delusions ('myxoedema madness').

Cretinism is the name sometimes given to hypothyroidism occurring in newborn babies whose thyroid gland fails to develop. Unless diagnosed and treated within a matter of weeks, the child will remain permanently dwarfed and mentally retarded (a cretin), so the condition should be suspected in all babies who are small, fail to feed well or are rather sluggish and underactive. Points to look for are the rather yellow complexion caused by carotene in the skin, a large, protruding tongue and umbilical hernia.

THE ADRENAL GLANDS

These glands are actually double glands, one inside the other, each arising from different embryonic tissue. The central part, the medulla, derives from nervous tissue and secretes the hormones adrenalin and noradrenalin. It seldom malfunctions except in the very rare instance of a benign tumor secreting these substances in excess, called a 'phaeochromocytoma' (Gr.phaeos = grey; chromos = colour; cytos = cell). This causes paroxysms of sweating, palpitations, headache and hypertension along with a degree of panic from the rush of adrenalin. However, it is more commonly the cortex which malfunctions, either over or underproducing the hormone cortisone and leading to Cushing's syndrome or Addison's disease respectively (although both of these are rare).

Cushing's syndrome is a collection of symptoms arising from an excess of circulating steroid hormones in the body and is most commonly iatrogenic in origin when it is seen in those being treated with long-term cortisone for asthma, rheumatoid arthritis or one of the collagen diseases. It may also be caused by a tumour in the cortex stimulating overproduction of steroid hormones, or even in the pituitary causing excess ACTH secretion.

Whatever the cause, the symptoms are seen first in the face which becomes rounded and moon-shaped, while the skin becomes discoloured and reddened with a degree of acne. The trunk also swells and stretch marks and bruises appear on the skin, very like those seen during pregnancy. The fat over the shoulders increases and the bones become thin and brittle, especially those of the spine which starts to collapse, leading to the familiar 'buffalo hump'. There is usually a rise in blood pressure, and because cortisone mobilises glucose from the cells of the liver, glycosuria appears.

It is only a minority of those treated with cortisone who develop this syndrome, for it is related to the dosage of the drug as well as the duration of use. Except in young babies, cortisone cream applied to the skin will not cause internal effects, nor will that inhaled for asthma in aerosols or injected into joints in arthritis. However anyone on steroids taken systemically must be weaned off them with extreme care, as their own adrenal cortex will be suppressed from lack of ACTH, so they are totally dependent on an external supply to protect them from going into 'acute adrenal failure'.

Addison's disease is the opposite condition to Cushing's, for here the body has effectively run out of hydrocortisone, which is required for protection against stress. It may arise from destruction of the adrenal cortex by tumour, including metastatic cancers, from TB, or more commonly from an autoimmune process similar to that of Hashimoto's disease in the thyroid, and indeed the two sometimes coincide. The symptoms are essentially the reverse of those of hyperadrenalism – weakness, low blood pressure, loss of weight and hypoglycaemia leading eventually to coma. There is often a darkening of the skin with pigmentation especially of the nipples and the inside of the cheeks if the disease has been gradually progressing for a long time.

DIABETES MELLITUS

The pancreas has already featured in the digestive disorders, but here we are interested in the more common consequence of pancreatic dysfunction – diabetes mellitus (not to be confused with diabetes insipidus, an entirely unrelated disorder). Diabetes mellitus (L.mellis = sweet) occurs as a result of diminution or absence of insulin supplied by the beta cells of the Islets of Langerhans. Complete and rapid atrophy of these cells is more likely to come about in children and adolescents and lead suddenly to what is termed *juvenile-onset diabetes*.

In the middle-aged and elderly, however, diabetes usually results from an insufficient quantity of insulin for the amount of tissue it has to supply, and so arises when there is either an excessive amount of tissue, i.e. obesity, or when the pancreas has only partially failed, the condition being known as *maturity-onset diabetes*. Obviously the former cases will require insulin, which must be taken in the form of an injection as, being

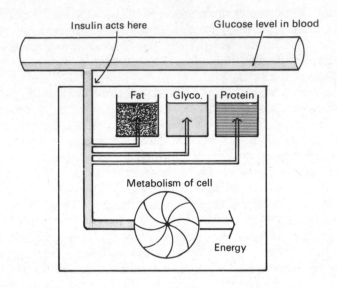

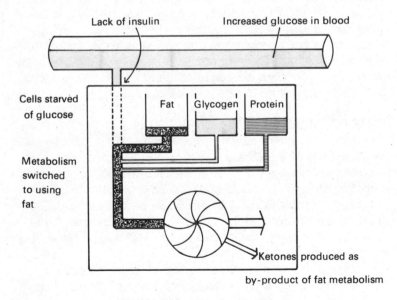

FIGURE 16.1   *Cellular metabolism of glucose in A. normal and B. diabetic*

a protein, it is rapidly destroyed by the secretions of the stomach. The latter type, the maturity onset diabetics, are usually able to stabilise their blood sugar on diet alone or with the addition of anti-diabetic drugs to stimulate the beta cells.

The cause of the atrophy of the beta-cells is in the majority of cases unknown, but destruction by an autoimmune process is highly likely. In a very small percentage of cases the pancreas is damaged by a tumour or pancreatitis. Certainly there is an increased risk of the condition among the relatives of those who suffer from it, and among those of Jewish extraction, indicating a genetic component in the aetiology.

The symptomatology of the types is rather different. Juvenile-onset diabetics are seen less frequently but the onset is fairly rapid over a few days or weeks, and is often precipitated by an illness or infection. Because one of the main roles of insulin is in regulating the flow of glucose from the blood into the cells, there will be a feeling of weakness and poor appetite as glucose is unable to enter the cells and build up in the blood leading to *hyperglycaemia*. Once it reaches a certain level it can no longer be retained by the kidney and overflows into the urine as *glycosuria*, taking with it considerable quantities of water to carry it, so *polyuria* and *nocturia* develop. To compensate for this the patient becomes *thirsty* and drinks more, often craving sweet things, as the cells are deprived of sugar. The glycosuria may lead to *infections* developing such as cystitis, balanitis and pruritus vulvae, while the increase in glucose in the aqueous humour of the eye can increase the refractive index and alter the vision to cause blurring and difficulty focussing.

The sudden disappearance of insulin from the scene in juvenile onset diabetes means that other arrangements have to be made to supply the cells with energy, and this comes in the form of fat which is taken from the body stores (see figure 16.1). The patient therefore starts to lose weight quite rapidly, but when the fat is used to create energy it also produces large quantities of acidic substances called *ketones* or *ketone bodies* which are toxic to the body and so are rapidly excreted by both the lungs and the kidney (*ketonuria*). By the time such a situation has been reached the patient is usually *dehydrated* from the glycosuria and ketonuria, and may become somewhat stuporose from the build-up of acids in the blood, or even eventually unconscious in *diabetic coma*. In order to rid the body of the ketones more rapidly, the respiratory centre is stimulated to breathe more deeply and quickly – *air hunger* or 'Kussmaul's breathing' – and acetone can be smelt on the breath. If insulin and intravenous fluids are not received the patient's condition is likely to deteriorate and before the advent of insulin was invariably fatal.

In maturity-onset diabetics such a dramatic turn of events is seldom seen as some insulin is present, and indeed many patients have no symptoms at all and their diabetes is only discovered on a routine urinalysis. So why, then, does it matter whether or not the condition is discovered? The answer is that over a number of years complications set in which can be greatly reduced if treatment is started early, and some maturity-onset diabetics can even present initially with symptoms of the complications. These include leg cramps, poor circulation, skin ulcers, infections, poor vision, tingling in the hands and feet and vague complaints such as apathy or tiredness.

Complications of Diabetes

Because diabetes is a condition which continues for the duration of a patient's life, there is an accumulation of side-effects which develop with time, although these can be minimized with effective control of the blood sugar. These are:

– *Atherosclerosis*, which occurs much more frequently because of the simultaneous disruption of fat metabolism in diabetics and increase in the circulating levels of cholesterol in the blood. This leads to intermittent claudication, gangrene and ulcers in the feet, as well as a greater likelihood of heart attacks, strokes and hypertension.

– *Infections* are especially common in diabetics. As well as those of the urinary tract mentioned, some diabetics are troubled with persistant skin infections, vaginitis and boils, while TB is also more common.

– *Peripheral neuropathy* is a disorder of the peripheral nerves caused by damage to their blood supply by the diabetes. The sensory nerves are most often affected with tingling (paraesthesiae) and numbness of the arms and legs, later followed by weakness and paralysis. If the autonomic nerves are affected then failure of erection and impotence may result, or persistant diarrhoea.

– *Renal disease.* A particular kind of lesion occurs in the glomerular capillaries of many diabetics whereby they become thickened, leading ultimately to chronic renal failure and uraemia. This complication is usually announced by the appearance in the urine of persistant proteinuria, but may take many years before complete failure ensues.

– *Retinopathy.* This is the commonest complication of young diabetics and leads to blindness in a small proportion. The retinal capillaries start to disintegrate and leak blood into the vitreous which causes scarring and distortion. As a result of the stimulus new capillaries may start to grow out into the vitreous and further obliterate vision, and it is these which are destroyed with the aid of a laser to preserve vision. As well as retinopathy, cataracts are slightly more common in diabetics.

TABLE 16.1   Possible causes of weight loss

Condition	Pointers
Depression/anxiety	Stressful life situation
Anorexia nervosa	Amenorrhoea, induced vomiting, constipation, hair loss
Malabsorption	Cystic fibrosis, coeliac disease, Crohn's, ulcerative
Travel	Parasitic gut infection, hepatitis, poor food
Alcoholism	Insomnia, tremor, blackouts, memory lapses
Chronic fever	Hepatitis, RA, glandular fever, polymyalgia rheumatica
Peptic ulcer	Pain, vomiting, history
Tuberculosis	Cough, night sweats
Diabetes mellitus	Polyuria, thirst, dizziness, sugar craving
Hyperthyroidism	Hyperactive, hot, sweating, diarrhoea, palpitations
Cancer	Usually only when secondaries, unless stomach involved
Renal disease	Nocturia, frothy urine, oedema

Treatment of Diabetes

The object of all diabetic treatment is to maintain the blood glucose at as near a normal level as possible. By doing so the short and long term complications are avoided and one can live a virtually normal life, subject only to the inconvenience of having to carry around such things as syringes, urinalysis tablets and in some cases blood glucose analysis apparatus. The basic way of measuring one's blood glucose is still by examining the urine and making the assumption that if it is glucose-free then there is no excess in the blood. However, this is not always the case, nor does it inform the patient when their glucose is falling to a dangerously low level. So nowadays more sophisticated methods are applied, such as taking a drop of blood and examining the colour change when it is applied to a chemically treated paper, which gives a direct and instantaneous result and can be performed by the diabetic himself. Under experimental trial is an 'electronic pancreas' which will analyse blood glucose and automatically inject the correct dose.

Insulin is usually necessary for juvenile-onset diabetics, who are thus also known as *insulin dependent* diabetics. This is normally injected once or twice a day just before a meal, and as different types of insulin are released at different rates into the blood, by mixing them in a single morning dose it is possible to supply the body continually throughout the next 24 hours with only minor fluctuations in the blood level. This does, of course, depend on a very steady and regular intake of food, and if meals are missed then problems can arise. It also depends on a regular level of activity, for if extra physical work is done then both more glucose and more insulin will be required, so if a diabetic wishes to lead an active and varied life, they must be conversant with the mechanism of insulin treatment and diet. Much of the work of diabetic clinics is spent in education for diabetes, as well as checking for side effects of the disease and regulating blood sugar levels. The latter is done in two ways, once by examining the patient's chart of their urinalsis over a daily or weekly basis, or by analysing what is called their glycosylated haemoglobin.

During the life of a red cell the haemoglobin is exposed to the fluctuating levels of blood glucose over that period, and this glucose attaches itself to haemoglobin A1c especially and forms glycosylated haemoglobin. The percentage of glycosylated haemoglobin in the blood thus gives a faily good measure of the prevailing levels of glucose over the previous three months, and should normally be below 8%. If it is substantially greater than this figure, it indicates that blood glucose has been consistantly high and the treatment needs a review.

Some diabetics, however carefully they try to control their blood sugar level, find that it oscillates wildly up and down no matter how they regulate their diet and insulin, and they are sometimes termed *brittle diabetics*. This happens particularly during pregnancy in some women, because the sex hormones cause a certain resistance to insulin. If the blood glucose descends below a certain level the symptoms of *hypoglycaemia* develop – sweating, weakness, palpitations, tremor and eventually confusion and coma. In a minority such events may happen with dramatic suddenness, and are known as *insulin comas*. Such episodes are more likely if a meal is late or missed, and are also caused by even quite small amounts of alcohol, so diabetics should always carry an emergency supply of glucose tablets. One of the problems which sometimes occurs in the treatment of diabetics is to decide whether their unconsciousness is due to diabetic or insulin coma, for the treatment is completely different, and to give too much insulin is very dangerous, so if there is doubt it is better to give glucose.

Diet is necessary for all diabetics, both in order to lose weight so as to conserve the existing supplies of insulin, and in order to balance the quantity of injected insulin. In most maturity-onset diabetics diet alone will clear the urine of glucose, and enable them to lose weight where necessary. But sometimes the assistance of so-called *hypoglycaemic drugs* which act on the pancreas is needed. About one third of diabetics take them, and they stimulate the pancreas to release greater quantities of insulin. However, in the event of an acute illness such as influenza, there may be a need to introduce injections of insulin for a while especially if there is vomiting.

CHAPTER SEVENTEEN

BRAIN:
DISORDERS OF
COMMUNICATION

*T*he nervous system consists broadly of two parts, a central area for the storage, retrieval and coordination of information – the brain and spinal cord, and a peripheral nervous system consisting of sensory, motor and autonomic nerves which gather information and execute instructions. The central and peripheral nervous systems have a considerable degree of overlap, but because the former is contained wholly within the bony confines of the skull and spinal cord, it is vulnerable to changes in pressure which may arise, since there is little room for expansion. Disorders of the central nervous system are discussed in this chapter, the main ones being vascular problems, infections, tumours, functional disorders such as migraine and epilepsy and various types of degeneration.

STROKES

The term aptly describes a condition of the brain characterised by its abrupt onset and widespread and often devastating effects. The name derives from the old fashioned word *apoplexy*, which comes from the Greek meaning 'to be struck down', and the current medical term of *cerebro-vascular accident* or CVA indicates that the underlying pathological basis is a vascular disorder. The brain demands the major share of cardiac output as it is especially vulnerable to oxygen lack, and it is well supplied by two pairs of arteries which link together at its base to form the circle of Willis. This arrangement enables blood flow to be restored in the event of one artery failing, and from this circle a number of branches penetrate the brain. However these are particularly liable to *atherosclerosis* and its attendant complications of *haemorrhage, embolism* and *thrombosis*.

Depending on the particular artery affected, the symptoms of a stroke will vary and may cover a wide range, from visual disturbance and dizziness to paralysis, confusion and anaesthesia. Because of the decussation of nerve fibres, any weakness or anaesthesia will be on the side of the body opposite to that of the stroke and the nature of the symptoms will give a clue to the location of the lesion in the brain. For instance, if the whole of one side is paralysed – a *hemiplegia* – then it is probable that the infarcted area was supplied by the middle cerebral artery, whereas when the posterior artery is involved then it is the occipital lobe and consequently sight which is affected.

The speed and manner of the onset of symptoms may also give a clue to the nature of the underlying pathology. Strokes often occur at night, when the flow is most sluggish and prone to thrombosis, and it is not uncommon for an elderly person to wake with symptoms, and at one time young women who took oral contraceptives with larger quantities of oestrogens than are used today were also at slight risk. When a CVA occurs during exercise, especially in someone who is known to be hypertensive, it is likely to be the result of haemorrhage from one of the cerebral arteries. This may also occur outside the brain, in the meninges (see below). Occasionally a stroke may 'evolve' over a period of several days, and there will be a progressive increase in disability.

Who, then, is at risk from strokes? By and large strokes occur more in women than in men and particularly among those with *hypertension* or *diabetes* or in fact any condition which leads to atherosclerosis such as smoking and familial hypercholesterolaemia. The incidence in the over 65s is relatively high, about one in 500, and this makes it the commonest cause of death after coronary heart disease and cancer. However one person in three who gets a stroke will recover more or less completely in time, so the prognosis is by no means uniformly poor. Occasionally young people are at risk from a CVA because they develop malignant hypertension or even a tumour.

If the cause is an embolus, this will often arise in an area of atherosclerosis which may be distant from the brain, or in the wall of the heart following an infarction (mural thrombus). If the embolus is small or composed only of platelets it may be quickly broken up by the flow of blood, so the symptoms are only transient and the episode is referred to as a *transient ischaemic attack* (TIA). Such attacks sometimes cause a temporary episode of confusion or unconsciousness, or may involve the visual cortex and lead to the symptom of *amaurosis* (temporary blindness) with the sense of a curtain being drawn across the visual field. Sometimes there may be a transient hemiplegia or *dysphasia* (loss of speech) lasting minutes or hours and then recovering. A TIA is often an advance warning that a major stroke could happen within a few months.

Not all cerebral ischaemia results in strokes, for if the flow of blood is very gradual, as is sometimes the case, then the brain will progressively atrophy and lead to a general loss of intellectual function and memory. This *diffuse cerebral atherosclerosis* is reflected in an increasing degree of *dementia* and may be presaged by emotional liability and apathy. As a cause of senile dementia it is much less common than Alzheimer's disease (see below), but the two can sometimes be difficult to distinguish from one another.

SUBARACHNOID HAEMORRHAGE

Just as haemorrhage can occur within the brain tissue in the form of intracerebral haemorrhage mentioned above, so it may occur under or between the coverings of the brain, the meninges, and is known variously as subarachnoid, subdural or extradural depending on the exact location.

Of these the commonest is a *subarachnoid haemorrhage*, where blood leaks into the space beneath the arachnoid layer normally occupied by the CSF, and this usually derives from the rupture of a congenital defect of the circle of Willis which takes the form of a *berry aneurysm*. The composer Mendelssohn died at the age of 38 from just such a cause, as did his sister, father and grandfather, and it is notable that he complained of severe headaches for months before he succumbed, when the aneurysm was slowly leaking. This is the main symptom and is described as a stiffness in the neck, sometimes coming on very suddenly and accompanied by photophobia, nausea, dizziness and even loss of consciousness. The young and middle-aged are particularly affected, more often women, and those with hypertension are especially susceptible. If there is doubt about the diagnosis then examination of the CSF by lumbar puncture will show bloodstained fluid, and if necessary an Xray of the vessels of the brain incorporating contrast medium (angiogram) will show the exact position of the leak, which may require an operation to tie it off.

Subdural haemorrhage develops, as the name suggests, beneath the dura and is seen mostly in the very young and the elderly. It is liable to occur in babies born prematurely, for in them the skull is still relatively soft and allows damage to the veins which cross the subdural space. Such infants may become permanently brain-damaged by such a bleed, and this is one reason for the application of forceps – to protect the head from compression during birth. In the elderly a subdural haemorrhage may follow a mild blow to the head, and it may take many weeks for the symptoms to manifest fully. There is a slow leakage of blood which gradually compresses the brain tissue and leads to drowsiness, weakness, confusion and headaches, and this can be put down to senility while the original blow has been forgotten. An operation to remove the collecting clot of blood may be needed to remove the pressure and restore normality.

Extradural haemorrhage arises from a head injury which ruptures the outermost vessels and causes a substantial bleed, resulting in symptoms soon after the injury. These will vary with the severity of the trauma, the

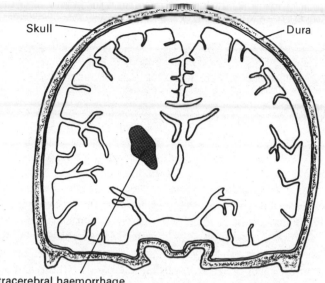

Skull — Dura

Intracerebral haemorrhage

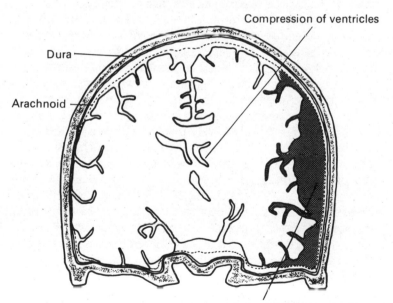

Compression of ventricles

Dura —

Arachnoid —

Subarachnoid haemorrhage

FIGURE 17.1   *Cross section of brain to show A. Intracerebral haemorrage (stroke), and B. subarachnoid haemorrhage*

most mild being a severe headache, nausea and vomiting, but sometimes progressing quickly to loss of consciousness or deep coma. It is this condition which should be remembered in someone who might appear to be drunk and involved in a fight or road accident, but who may only have a few hours to live if their condition is not treated surgically.

MENINGITIS

The central nervous system is usually well insulated from most infections, because it possesses a barrier in the form of the meninges, and the only route in is via the bloodstream unless the skull is fractured. Meningitis is the most common of the infections of the brain, but the deeper tissues may be affected in encephalitis, and sometimes a local infection can spread as an abscess from a neighbouring structure such as the middle ear.

Meningitis, which is an infection of the cerebrospinal fluid with inflammation of the meninges, can be either viral or bacterial (or very rarely amoebic) in origin. The word *meningism* is used to describe the characteristic stiffness of the neck which is a feature, but this is also seen in subarachnoid haemorrhage and in children with high fevers such as tonsillitis. Meningitis is most common in children, and many if not most cases are of viral origin, particularly mumps and the enteroviruses. Bacterial meningitis is often meningococcal and occurs in epidemics, especially in parts of Africa where it can be spread by insects. In the UK meningococcal meningitis is spread by droplet infection, often through carriers who have no symptoms themselves and who number about 10% of the population. Young children have not developed any immunity to the disease and if they are susceptible may incubate it in their nasal passages for a few days before it spreads via the blood to other parts of the body.

The spread through *septicaemia* is sudden and sometimes over-whelming, perhaps leading rapidly to widespread bleeding into the skin with coma and usually death within 24 hrs, and it is this form of the disease which has given meningitis its fearful reputation. Most cases advance less rapidly, though, and develop fever, headache, stiff neck, photophobia and then a rose-red rash on the buttocks and thighs. In younger children the diagnosis may be especially difficult as the symptoms are less specific, and the only certain way of excluding the possibility is to remove some CSF by lumbar puncture. The possible routes which the course of the disease can take is illustrated in table 17.1.

Recently other forms of meningitis have come into the picture, such as those caused by other bacteria, particularly E. coli, streptococci and Listeria. The latter is a very common bacillus, and can be found in the soil, water, food (especially soft cheese) and even sometimes as a vaginal

TABLE 17.1   The possible consequences of meningococcal infection

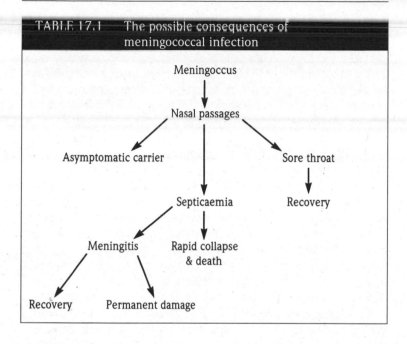

commensal. *Listeriosis* is liable to cause damage to the foetus if contracted by the mother during pregnancy, when it is often unrecognised as she may only suffer a very mild illness, whereas the baby can contract pneumonia at around the time of birth, or meningitis some weeks later.

Another uncommon form of meningitis is the tuberculous variety, seen in undernourished children but fortunately no longer common in this country. It starts slowly and insidiously but progresses inexorably to leave a thick exudate on the meninges which causes severe headache and paralysis. The spread occurs in the bloodstream, usually originating soon after the primary focus has established itself in the lung and before there are any symptoms there.

Encephalitis is almost invariably a viral infection and may accompany many of the more common viral illnesses such as influenza, mumps and glandular fever, in which it is the cause of the severe headache and drowsiness. Occasionally, however, the condition progresses to other symptoms – fits, paralysis or coma, and may lead to lasting damage. Some cases of Parkinsonism are attributable to previous attack by encephalitis lethargica virus of which there was a world-wide pandemic shortly after the First World War. More recently a form of encephalitis has been noted to occur in AIDS patients and leads to the cerebral symptoms which are part of the terminal picture (see chapter 2).

Cerebral abscess is a type of infection not often seen, caused by the local spread of infection through the skull and from a focus usually in the middle ear or sinuses, or sometimes from a more distant blood-borne site. As the abscess expands it causes symptoms from pressure, such as headache, nausea and vomiting, but is also accompanied by fever and later paralysis or weakness.

MYALGIC ENCEPHALOMYELITIS (ME)

Few diseases have been so misunderstood or so maligned as ME, perhaps because it so often resembles other conditions, and because there appear to be as yet few tests which can 'prove' the diagnosis. As the name suggests, the foremost symptom is that of muscular pain and stiffness, as well as the very profound fatigue which is almost universal. The fact that these effects are felt most severely by those who were previously most active, as well as its prevalence in the young, especially those aged between 10 and 30, has led to the rather unfortunate name of 'yuppie flu'.

ME is now thought to be a variety of viral encephalitis, and occurs both sporadically and in epidemics, of which one of the most renowned is that which affected the staff (but not the patients) of the Royal Free Hospital in 1955. Subsequent allegations of 'mass hysteria' attached an unfair assumption that it was a psychosomatic condition, but there is now much evidence to incriminate a virus and any psychological sequelae, especially the very common depression and panic attacks, are a result rather than a cause. Other features of the disease are swollen glands, a persistent headache, numbness and paraesthesia in the extremities ('glove and stocking anaesthesia'), muscle twitching and a sore throat. Less commonly a fever, shortness of breath and diarrhoea are felt, and there may be pain in the chest which can mimic a heart attack.

After a week or two of acute symptoms there follows a prolonged period of recovery which is very variable and may range from one to more than thirty years. During this time there is great fatigueability of muscles, and the least effort is rewarded with profound exhaustion and inability to concentrate so that even reading becomes difficult. Complete rest is therefore essential, although insomnia is often a problem. Some find that they are affected by a particular food which may exacerbate the symptoms and they learn to avoid it. All in all there is daily variation in the symptoms, and even from month to month, for instance in women who tend to have a premenstrual relapse.

Medical research into ME has tended in two directions, metabolic and viral. Because the pancreas plays a vital role in the maintenance of the glucose and hence the energy within the body, and because many ME sufferers are found to be hypoglycaemic periodically as well as developing symptoms after meals, it is possible that this organ is a target for damage. Whether this is in the form of a direct viral assault or indirectly from an auto-immune pathology is open to speculation at present. Another metabolic possibility is that the neurological damage leaves an imbalance of certain neurotransmitters which results in abnormal muscle metabolism on exercise.

What does seem certain is that the initial phase of the illness is the result of an infective process, probably associated with either the Coxsackie virus (another strain of which is responsible for Bornholm disease) or with the polio virus, as antibodies to either of these are seen in the blood. It may be that in certain individuals one of these causes damage to the immune system which in turn leads to malfunctioning of the body's metabolism. It is not uncommon for many viral infections to lead to 'post-viral fatigue' and ME may simply be an extreme version of this.

HEADACHE

Strange as it may seem there are no sensory receptors in the brain itself, so this extremely common symptom is almost always caused by pressure on the meninges or tension in the muscles rather than intracerebral pathology, but it is obviously important to exclude the latter. So-called *tension headaches* are a result of chronic contraction of the muscles of the neck (from withdrawal and fear) or of the scalp and around the eyes (grief and sadness). They are therefore characterised by being felt as a tightness of the neck or eyes, increasing as the day wears on but usually alleviated by sleep.

Migraine is a very common form of headache, and susceptibility to it runs in families, but here the term specifically indicates a headache caused by alteration of the size of the vessels in the brain. This can come about from stress or from hormonal changes as occurs around the period, from the contraceptive pill or following the consumption of certain foods, particularly milk, eggs, cheese, chocolate, oranges, tomatoes, alcohol and some additives such as tartrazine.

The symptoms of migraine are only too well known to those who suffer from them, and attacks usually start with distorted vision and flashing lights, coloured zig-zag lines across the field of vision (*fortification spectra*), *difficulty focussing* and *photophobia*. These are caused by an initial contraction of vessels in the visual cortex, which later expand to cause the characteristic throbbing, bursting sensation lasting sometimes for hours. If the attack is severe, there may also be tingling and numbness, often around the mouth, but sometimes involving a limb and even causing temporary paralysis. The headache usually starts on one side of the head (*hemicrania*) and is accompanied by nausea, vomiting and sometimes diarrhoea.

Certain variations of classical migraine occur, including *cluster headaches* which are typically severe, neuralgic pains situated around the eye and occurring in clusters every few weeks or months, then disappearing completely in between. They are often accompanied by redness and watering of the eye and perhaps a nasal discharge also. Some children develop recurrent abdominal pain and vomiting which has a certain similarity to migraine and is therefore sometimes known as *abdominal migraine*. Certainly there is a higher than average incidence of migrainous headaches in later life.

Orthodox treatment for migraine uses drugs containing ergotamine, a drug which constricts the vessels and thus counteracts the dilation which causes the headache, sometimes with the addition of an antiemetic. These drugs are sometimes given in the form of suppositories for speed of action, but an excessive amount will lead to Raynaud's phenomenon (see chapter 10).

Raised intracranial pressure is a term used to describe a situation resulting from a variety of causes such as *malignant hypertension*, *brain tumour* and *abscess*, and which leads to a characteristic occipital pain which is worst on rising in the morning but tends to improve with upright posture as the day progresses. It is a persistent pain, made worse by any kind of straining, bending or coughing which increase the pressure of the CSF, and often accompanied by sudden vomiting without nausea owing to direct stimulation of the vomiting centre. There may also be accompanying visual disturbance or diplopia with dizziness from pressure on sensitive areas, and epileptic fits may occur in the case of intracranial tumours. A similar type of pain caused by meningeal irritation is seen in meningitis as already mentioned, and also following a lumbar puncture due to the sudden lowering of the pressure of the cerebrospinal fluid.

Not all headaches are a result of meningeal or vascular stimulation, and the possibility of referred pain in the head from a neighbouring structure must be born in mind, particularly the eyes, sinuses, cranial nerves and cervical spine. *Glaucoma* is an uncommon but elusive pain, being transmitted to the head, face or even abdomen. *Sinusitis* will mostly exhibit tenderness of the relevant area, while neuralgia of the cranial nerves is characteristic. *Trigeminal neuralgia* is the usual culprit, less often the glossopharyngeal nerve, and the pain is sudden, severe and lancinating, often being stimulated by chewing or touching the affected part, and radiating over the area supplied by the lower parts of the trigeminal nerve. *Tic douloureux* is the alternative name, and it is a condition of elderly people unless it represents an early symptom of multiple sclerosis which it may rarely do in the young. Pain in the upper division of the nerve is usually the first evidence of herpes zoster or *shingles* (q.v.) as this is its preferred site.

TABLE 17.1	Possible causes of headache
Condition	**Pointers**
Tension/anxiety	Band-like, worse evenings
Depression	Frontal, weepy, bereaved
Pyrexial	Especially viral infections
Dehydration	Especially if alcohol induced
Hypoglycaemia	Sometimes related to meals
Migraine	Visual disturbance, nausea, photophobia
Post-traumatic	History of concussion
Meningitis	Sudden, fever, photophobia, neck stiffness
Cluster headache	History, eye may water
Cervical spondylosis	Occipital, related to movement
Hyptertension	Only if severe
Temporal arteritis	Age, weight loss, malaise, visual involvement
Raised intracranial pressure	Vomiting, photophobia, continuous, severe
Paget's disease	Enlarging skull
Drug induced	Cough syrups, Indocid, the Pill, digitalis
Extracranial	Glaucoma, sinusitis, trigeminal neuralgia

EPILEPSY

There are 100,000 million nerve cells in the brain, each with the potential to be switched either in the 'on' position or the 'off', so it is not at all surprising that on occasions a cell gets overexcitable and triggers a wave of impulses which sweep across large areas causing havoc. The outward signs are of a body which has been seized by some external force, and this is what gives epilepsy its name, from the Greek word epilepto meaning 'seize hold'. Strictly speaking epilepsy is a symptom rather than a disease, and the word gives no clue as to the underlying pathology but is merely a description. The various types of epilepsy simply indicate the origin and course of the electrical impulses involved.

Most of us have experienced an occasional twitching of a muscle, known as *myoclonus*, often involving the muscles in the eyelid or face or thumb. Sometimes, just at the moment of drifting off to sleep, the whole body may give an involuntary jerk. These occur because the normal inhibition of impulse discharge is lost by some neurones, and as the cortex devotes proportionately more motor neurones to control of the face and hands, it is therefore more likely for one of these to be the site of origin. If the discharge were to take place in the temporal lobe, then the result would be a more subjective phenomenon, such as is described below.

About 1 person in 200 suffers from some ongoing form of epilepsy which requires treatment, and there is a tendency for it to run in families. Many people, however, have a single fit at some time in their lives, especially during childhood when the CNS is more easily stimulated, but one one must be careful about using the diagnosis 'epileptic' on them because it is a difficult one to lose, and once drug treatment has been started there may be a reluctance to discontinue it.

In any form of repetitive seizure there is always a group of abnormal cells given to paroxysmal discharge, and the form which the seizure takes will depend first on their location and second on the pathway and pattern of spread of the discharge. If the focus remains in the part of the brain where it arises then a *partial seizure* is said to have occurred, and this is the type of which *temporal lobe* epilepsy is an example. On occasions the outer limits of this partial seizure will touch upon the deeper structures of the brain and be followed by spread to a secondary *generalised seizure*, which is that characterised by *grand mal* epilepsy (see below). The third type illustrated is where a discharge is initiated in the central parts of the brain and spreads to affect consciousness, which may quickly recover as in *petit mal*, or be lost for some time as in some types of grand mal. Each of these types of fit may, or may not, exhibit an abnormal discharge when measured on the electroencephalogram (EEG) in between events, and this can be useful as evidence in making a diagnosis.

Epilepsy arising for the first time in an adult is always a rather suspicious sign that some serious underlying condition such as a tumour or abscess or even dementia has arisen. Sometimes there is an obvious underlying cause such as a stroke, meningitis or head injury, and such problems as alcoholism and drug taking are associated with a much higher incidence of epilepsy. Babies, especially if premature, may suffer from epilepsy at the time of birth due to hypoglycaemia or anoxia, and sometimes from an excessive quantity of calcium obtained from early feeding with cow's milk. In childhood, *febrile convulsions* are very common during a cold or other fever and these are mentioned in more detail below, along with the other major types of epilepsy.

Grand mal epilepsy is a form of generalised seizure where

consciousness is lost for a time, and may arise from either an extension from a partial seizure, in which case the first phase will be prominent, or arise *de novo* from a primary generalised seizure. The convulsions may be repeated, sometimes several times a day, and usually exhibit four separate but consecutive stages:

– *The aura*, during which the person will have a premonition that an attack is about to happen, and which is felt either as a change in mood some days before, or perhaps as a definite sensation only a few seconds or minutes prior to the attack. It could be a smell, a sound, a tingling sensation or even a sense of deja vu, of having been here before, but is the same on each occasion.

– *The tonic phase* is when unconsciousness occurs and the person suddenly contracts their muscles and becomes rigid, often with a cry or a grunt. They will fall to the ground and stop breathing temporarily so become slightly blue, and may bit their lip or tongue, or perhaps void urine.

– *The clonic phase* then follows, which consists of jerking, convulsive movements (clonus) of the whole body, which lasts a few minutes and is accompanied by heavy stertorous breathing and sometimes frothing at the mouth. This then passes into the last or

– *The relaxation phase*, when a stuporose, confused and very sleepy state supervenes followed by a gradual return to full consciousness and the headache which frequently follows.

If there is a delay in coming out of the clonic phase and the patient remains continually twitching, a situation sometimes seen in drug withdrawal or head injuries, this is termed *status epilepticus* (c.f. status asthmaticus) and requires urgent treatment if a state of permanent neurological damage is to be avoided.

Petit mal is a milder form of epilepsy seen mostly in children who exhibit sudden lapses in lucidity which are very short-lived and last only a matter of seconds. This means that they can be easily missed, for the onset and termination are abrupt and posture is maintained throughout. There may be many brief attacks in a day, in which the child stops what she is doing, looks down and may grimace or flutter her eyelids before continuing as before. It is often associated with myoclonus on waking in the morning, with much twitching and broken crockery at the breakfast table. Petit mal is usually outgrown by the teens, although it may rarely become grand mal later.

Psychomotor or *temporal lobe epilepsy* is, as the name suggests, localised in the temporal lobe where memory and some sensations are coordinated. There is thus a disturbance in the content of consciousness rather than of consciousness itself, and this leads to a great variety of possible forms which the attack may take. There may be hallucinations of hearing, taste or sight, or sometimes dream-like states when automatic acts or untypical and even antisocial behaviour is exhibited, later completely forgotten.

Febrile convulsions are a very common type of fit seen in children up to the age of five when in the throes of a feverish illness. They represent a sudden increase in the susceptibility of the brain to excitation, and there is often a history of similar attacks in the family. The parents can be reassured that they seldom lead to persistent epilepsy later and that the attacks are unlikely to be harmful unless they become continuous. Nevertheless it is important to exclude an underlying condition, especially meningitis.

Drug treatment of epilepsy is sometimes a difficult decision, for the simple reason that once started there is a strong possibility of having to continue for a long time, if not for life. Having said this, the ability to control fits completely is essential, for the presence of even one or two a year leads to problems at work, with social relationships and perhaps most importantly with the ability to drive. The law says that epileptics are not permitted to drive unless they have been free of fits while awake for a continuous period of two years, and this has an implication for any attempt to wean someone off anti-epileptic drugs.

The function of anti-epileptic drugs is to render the neurones less excitable and assist the function of the inhibitory pathways of the CNS. The short-acting barbiturate phenobarbitone has been used for many years, but this has the disadvantage of making adults very sleepy and children hyperactive so it is no longer a drug of first choice, although it can be very effective in resistant cases. The benzodiazepines are proving their worth now in epilepsy instead of as tranquillisers, and diazepam (Valium) is a very safe and effective drug for both febrile convulsions in children and status epilepticus, given intravenously or into the rectum.

The two most popular long-term drugs are phenytoin (Epanutin) and sodium valproate (Epilim), but these must be taken with great regularity to ensure an adequate level in the blood. Unfortunately they both have unwanted effects, phenytoin causing swelling and overgrowth of the gums when taken for a long time, as well as acne and skin problems, so it should be avoided if possible among adolescents. Epilim is very effective in most cases of grand mal, but may cause drowsiness and dizziness and some people notice an increase in their hair loss.

MULTIPLE SCLEROSIS

The nerve fibres of the brain and spinal cord are enclosed within a white sheath made of a fatty substance called myelin, and without the presence of this they are unable to conduct either sensory or motor impulses. Multiple or, as it was once called, disseminated sclerosis is a disease characterised by *demyelination* of the nerves in a more or less random manner, so that its symptoms are correspondingly variable and diagnosis often made difficult. As the areas of demyelination heal there is corresponding atrophy or sclerosis of the nerves worst affected, but others regain their function, so that the disease proceeds in a stepwise fashion with acute episodes followed by partial recovery, but overall is usually progressive. However, it is also the case that the disease is very variable both in duration and rate of deterioration and depends to some extent on which functions of the body are mainly affected. Most of those who develop MS can expect to live their normal life expectancy, and certainly over half survive 30 years or more from the time of diagnosis.

The distribution of MS in the world is curious, some races such as the Chinese, Japanese and Eskimos being virtually immune, and those who live near the equator being relatively free of it, which might lead one to think of a possible genetic predisposition. Britain has one of the higher incidences of the disease, while those living in the Orkneys & Shetlands having a fivefold increase and the highest incidence worldwide. This appearance as pockets of illness would seem to support an infective cause, and the appearance of antibodies against a variety of viruses in the CSF indicates this. No specific virus has been implicated, but it is quite possible that MS is an altered reaction of brain tissue to a common virus such as measles or herpes, precipitated by genetic and immunological factors.

The first appearance of the disease is generally in the young or middle-aged, rather more women than men contracting it and numbering about one in 2000 in this country. The first symptoms are very variable, and the most common are listed below, but an initial attack is almost invariably followed by remission, which may be permanent with complete recovery. The remission lasts a variable period, the average being about 2 years, but if a relapse occurs then other symptoms will make themselves known. In a few, and especially if MS starts with optical neuritis (see below), the condition runs a relatively benign course and fades out after one or two relapses. There are many reported long term remissions, so one should never give up hope even after years of having the disease.

The initial symptoms most commonly seen are:

– transient tingling or numbness in an area of the body, lasting a few days and then clearing up. A whole limb or only a small area may be affected, and may be followed by increased sensitivity for a whole.

– weakness of a hand or foot causing unaccustomed clumsiness or a tendency to trip easily. At times this will start after hard exercise or a hot bath.

– strange sensations, such as distortion of one's body image, a floating senation or feeling that one's head is detached.

– profound fatigue, difficulty remembering things.

– unsteadiness or staggering (*ataxia*) of the whole body, due to involvement of the cerebellum, sometimes with nausea and vomiting.

– blurred vision due to involvement of the optic nerve (*optic* or *retrobulbar neuritis*).

– double vision due to damage to the nerves supplying the extrinsic muscles of the eye.

– slurred speech (*dysarthria*), with typically jerky syllables.

– tinnitus and loss of balance.

The usual story is for the earlier symptoms to partly or completely clear after a week or two, sometimes never to return but more often to reoccur months later in similar form, with additional features. These may include:

– difficulty voiding urine (retention) or incontinence of urine.

– shooting pains down the back.

– painful spasms in the limbs.

– emotional changes, either depression or more often a degree of euphoria.

The main long-term problems for MS sufferers are the lack of control of the bladder which leads to urinary infections, the difficulty with walking which may mean using a wheelchair and eventually total paralysis, death if it occurs being due to the chest or renal infections resulting from immobility.

PARKINSON'S DISEASE

In 1817 Dr Parkinson described a condition commonly seen in the elderly which was characterised by rigidity and tremor and to which he gave the name *paralysis agitans* or the 'shaking palsy'. It is one of the most frequently met neurological conditions, seen in about 1 in 400 of the population over the age of 65, and caused by a decrease in the amount of the neurotransmitter *dopamine* found in the *basal ganglia*, the area of the brain responsible for the coordination of movement. Most of the cases are due to either atherosclerosis or unknown degenerative changes, but very occasionally in younger individuals the disorder is a result of poisoning or encephalitis. A very similar condition results as a side-effect of drug treatment for schizophrenia.

The clinical features of the disorder fall into two main categories, *tremor* and *rigidity*. The tremor is very typical and takes the form of a slow, coarse, regular shaking of the fingers and limbs, producing a characteristic 'pill-rolling' movement of the thumb and forefinger. This disappears during voluntary movement and comes back at rest so is known as a *resting tremor*.

However, tremor is the least disabling aspect. What is more of a problem is the stiffness and poverty of movement which may develop, and which causes difficulty in initiating activities such as walking, although once started a repetitive action can be maintained but is done stiffly and awkwardly. This rigidness, as well as being painful, causes difficulty with things like fastening buttons and shoelaces, writing, swinging the arms when walking and even speaking smoothly and clearly. There is a slowing of all movements and the facial expression becomes stiff and masklike, the eyes seldom blink and the gait becomes a shuffle with a tendency to trip over. Other features sometimes seen are excessive salivation, tiredness and depression.

To distinguish Parkinsonism from other types of tremor is usually not difficult. The tremors of anxiety and hyperthyroidism are more rapid, and so-called 'senile tremor' is continuous and does not fluctuate, being more of a kind of 'ditheriness'. Tremor arising from cerebellar disorders, while also causing ataxia, becomes worse on voluntary movement rather than improving (*intentional tremor*). When the arm or leg of someone with Parkinsonism is moved passively the combination of tremor and stiffness causes the characteristic 'cogwheel phenomenon', but sometimes tremor is absent and the rigidness is then described as 'lead pipe rigidity' as the limb suddenly 'gives' once the rigidity is overcome.

Treatment of Parkinsonism depends on replacing the missing dopamine by giving L dopa in tablet form, which improves the rigidity but has a less marked effect of the tremor. It is often given in combination with a drug which inhibits the enzyme in the brain that is responsible for breaking down dopamine (Sinemet, Madopar). Unfortunately the drugs have side-effects in the form of nausea and vomiting, and sometimes cardiac arrhythmias, and also have a tendency to lose efficacy after two years or so.

ALZHEIMER'S DISEASE

From the age of about 20 onwards the cells in our brain begin to die at an increasing rate every day, and are not replaced. Fortunately we possess such an incredible number that the effect is not noticeable, and until well beyond middle age experience more than counterbalances the loss. There comes a point, however, when such faculties as memory begin to deteriorate and elderly people are notorious for forgetfulness of recent things while still being able to recount the past in great detail. In a minority other mental faculties such as intellect and recognition are lost, and they are then said to be developing *senile dementia*, or, if it occurs at an earlier age, *pre-senile dementia*.

Like most other organs, failure of the brain is sometimes due to a lack of blood supply from generalised atherosclerosis with ensuing cerebral atrophy; in others the dementia is of the type known as *multi-infarct dementia* when multiple small strokes gradually diminish cortical function over a period of months until a critical 10% of tissue is lost and symptoms become manifest. By far the majority, however, take the form of degeneration first described by a German physician in 1907 and which therefore takes his name – Alzheimer's disease. This has come to play an increasing role in the elderly as the proportion of their population grows with improving longevity, and there are now some 75,000 cases in the UK, with 1 person in 5 affected to some degree over the age of 80. This puts a tremendous strain on the health-care facilities, and also accounts for the fourth highest mortality rate (after heart disease, cancer and strokes).

The first symptoms of the disease are subtle and may be only a worsening of the expected memory impairment of age. Disorientation is common, and there may be lack of recognition either of relatives, of what behaviour is appropriate to a situation or even of the difference between night and day. There is often a marked change in the personality, and the person can become emotionally labile and change from being mild-mannered to quite aggressive and abusive. All these changes make them difficult to relate to, and as they are unable to cope alone with running a home some kind of care is essential. Terminally they may lose all contact with the world and become totally dependent on being dressed, fed and sheltered.

The changes which Alzheimer described in the brain tissue were twofold. The first was that the nerve endings in the cortex were abnormally thickened and contained plaques of proteins, and the second was the marked tangling of the nerve fibres, in fact the greater the degree of tangling the worse was the dementia. There is now some, but not conclusive, evidence that at the centre of the tangle is an excess of aluminium and this has been blamed for the disease. It is true that those on renal dialysis who have increased blood levels of aluminium are more likely to suffer eventually from Alzheimer's disease, and there is also evidence that the distribution matches the quantity of aluminium in the water. But the final answers to Alzheimer's are yet to be discovered and much research is needed here.

CHAPTER EIGHTEEN

NERVES:
DISORDERS OF
FEELING & MOVEMENT

*I*nterruption, pressure or damage to the peripheral nerves may be the cause of pain or weakness in parts of the body supplied by them, and although there is considerable overlap with the nerves of the central nervous system the distinction is nevertheless useful. In general, if the reflex arc is intact as judged by the tendon reflexes, then it is unlikely that the peripheral nerves are involved, and this is one of the main uses of the test.

ENTRAPMENT SYNDROMES

There are many places in the body where nerves run in restricted spaces and are thus liable to compression from neighbouring structures such as bones, ligaments or fibrous tissue. These 'entrapment syndromes' as they are termed are very common, and two of them, *sciatica* and *carpal tunnel syndrome*, have already been described.

Brachial neuralgia is the name given to the pains which develop in the arm if the nerve is stretched by carrying heavy weights or compressed by one of the discs in the cervical vertebrae which is misplaced. The initial symptoms are usually *paraesthesiae* (pins and needles) running down the arm, followed by shooting pains and weakness of the muscles in the hands with a tendency to drop things. The pains may be present when the neck is flexed or the head turned, and there will often be tenderness over the affected disc.

On occasions a similar pain is felt down the front of the thigh in overweight individuals after they have been walking or standing for a while. This is due to compression of the lateral cutaneous nerve of the thigh where it runs under the inguinal ligament, and goes by the name of 'meralgia paraesthetica'.

Another place in the leg where nerves are liable to entrapment is immediately below the head of the fibula, either after an injury or in those who kneel crosslegged with one leg tucked underneath them. There is numbness of the upper part of the foot or even weakness or dorsiflexion of the ankle and 'foot drop'.

PERIPHERAL NEUROPATHY

The peripheral nerves are also liable to more diffuse disease, arising either from interference to the blood vessels which supply them, or from direct poisoning by toxins or drugs, or in some instances to allergy. Usually the neuropathy is secondary to an established condition such as diabetes mellitus, alcoholism or vitamin deficiency, in which case it comes on gradually as 'neuralgic' pains in the limbs with weakness, and is sometimes referred to as 'polyneuritis'. Sometimes only a single nerve is involved and then a 'mononeuritis' is the result, most commonly seen in diabetics.

One somewhat notorious type of polyneuritis is a condition known as the *Guillian-Barre syndrome*. It very occasionally follows immunisation or acute viral infections such as glandular fever, measles and herpes infections, arriving about two weeks after the infection. A widespread outbreak in the USA followed the mass immunisation programme against influenza in 1976. The symptoms arrive rapidly, usually in the space of a few hours, with tingling and numbness which start in the hands and feet as a 'glove and stocking' symptom, and then progress up the limbs to the trunk. The muscles weaken and become quite tender, and if the attack is a severe one then assisted respiration may be required for the duration of the acute phase, although the patient remains fully conscious as the higher centres are not involved. After several weeks the slow recovery begins and may take six months or more before completed, but there is seldom any residual disability. The most likely cause of this strange affliction is an allergic reaction by the body to either the virus or to the immunisation.

SPINA BIFIDA

As the embryo develops in the first few weeks of life, the vertebrae and spinal cord are formed by an infolding of the outermost layer of tissues which unite together to become the 'neural tube'. In the case of spina bifida there is a *neural tube defect* (NTD) to a variable degree when the tissues fail to join, so either just the vertebrae remain divided ('spina bifida occulta'), or the whole of the spinal cord lies exposed, covered only by a thin membrane, and the nerves themselves are atrophied.

About one baby in every 700 is born with a degree of spina bifida sufficient to affect function, and recently it has been possible to diagnose the condition before birth with accuracy by sampling the amniotic fluid and examining the protein secreted by the exposed tube, *alpha foeto-protein*. Not only is this present in large quantities in the amniotic sac, but some circulates in the mother's blood and a fair estimation of the presence of NTD may be made from this. The lumbo-sacral region is the area most

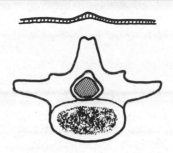

Normal development

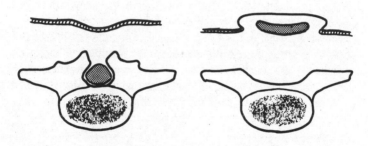

Occult spina bifida (symptomless)   Severe spina bifida

FIGURE 18.1   *Section through vertebrae showing position of spinal cord*
in neural tube defects

likely to be affected, and about one person in six has some evidence of a
slight failure of the vertebrae to fuse, shown by a small dimple with a tuft
of hair in it at the base of the spine.

Many possible causes have been proposed to account for spina bifida,
ranging from measles to the consumption of green potatoes in pregnancy,
but none have been substantiated even after extensive investigation.
Recent trials, however, have indicated that vitamin deficiency shortly
before and during pregnancy may be a factor, and supplements are
recommended for the first eight weeks. Mothers who take the anti-
epileptic drug Epilim may also be at an increased risk.

If a child is born with severe spina bifida it is the legs and bladder
which are most affected, with weakness and lack of sphincter control in

later life, leading to either retention or incontinence and frequent urinary infections. There may be impaired sensation to the legs and hence damage to the skin and subsequent ulceration. Men are liable to suffer from impotence because of the involvement of the nerves of erection, and this should be considered as a possible cause when investigating this condition.

If the spina bifida at birth is large and exposed to the air, then a decision must be made within a day or so as to whether to operate and close it, for otherwise infection to the cord and meningitis is a real risk. Many babies with severe NTD have an associated *hydrocephalus* on account of a blockage to the aqueduct leading out of the ventricles of the brain.

BELL'S PALSY

This is a condition of the seventh cranial nerve, the one which supplies the muscles of facial expression and taste. The nerve happens to run within a narrow bony canal at the point where it exits from the middle ear, and sometimes swells if the ear is exposed to a draught for a long period, or following an ear infection. Because it is unable to expand the oedema will prevent impulses passing down to the face which consequently becomes paralysed on one side. Thus the brow droops down and the person is

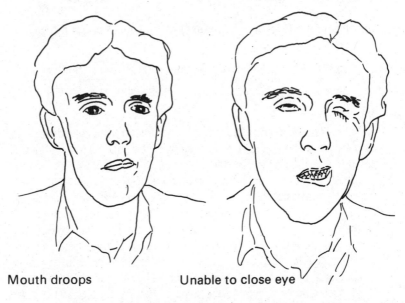

Mouth droops   **Unable to close eye**

FIGURE 18.2   *Right sided Bell's palsy A. with face relaxed, and B. on grimacing*

unable to close their eye which rolls up under the lid, nor can they frown or smile. The mouth sags and may cause slight dribbling, and tears will flow from the weakened eyelids. Sometimes there will be some loss of taste, and noises may be heard very intensely as the stapedius muscle in the ear, which normally dampens loud sounds, is put of action. Over half of those with Bell's palsy recover fully in 6 weeks or so and most of the remainder are left with only a minor disability.

POLIOMYELITIS

Since the immunisation programme in the UK in the early 50s polio has become a rare disease in this country, but it is still endemic in most third world countries and virtually all children there will have had contact with the virus. This is usually passed by the faecal-oral route in a manner similar to that of hepatitis A, but additionally an active case of polio, where there are sometimes flu-like symptons, can pass the virus by droplet infection.

Those who become infected usually develop no symptoms at all and are unaware that they have caught a potentially lethal disease, but about 1 in 10 have a slight fever and cough, and 1 in 50 contract the meningitis which usually results in paralysis of some degree. The latter develop the classical signs of meningism with stiff neck, headache and photophobia, and go on to get painful spasms in the limbs which then become partially paralysed. Because the anterior horn cells of the spinal cord are destroyed by the virus, there is a flaccid paralysis but no loss of sensation. In a severe case the upper part of the spine is also involved with paralysis of swallowing, breathing or speech and this carries a high mortality. If the patient survives, the paralysis improves to some degree with time, especially if they receive adequate physiotherapy, but some muscle wasting and weakness will be left in the limb.

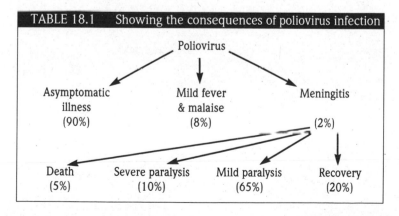

TABLE 18.1   Showing the consequences of poliovirus infection

Because of the prevalence of the virus among the populations of unimmunised countries, it is highly likely that those travelling there will come into contact with the disease, and immunisation should be very seriously considered. This is usually given as an attenuated form of the virus, the Sabin-type vaccine, and is taken orally. Because the virus is live, there is a very small risk, estimated at one in 4 million, of developing a paralytic illness of variable severity within a few weeks, and this can be avoided by having three injections of the Salk vaccine instead, which is a killed preparation.

CHAPTER NINETEEN

EYES: DISORDERS OF VISION

Vision is the sense which we can project over the furthest distance, literally beyond the stars, by making use of certain frequencies of electromagnetic radiation we call light. With this sense we can perceive danger at a much greater distance than sound or touch, but it has two drawbacks – the source must be in a direct line of vision, and there must be sufficient light reflected from the source, which means that during the hours of nightfall a somewhat different mechanism must operate. Because light waves do not travel round corners, our eyes must therefore be extremely mobile, and the best solution lies in a ball and socket arrangement, so the eyeball is normally a perfect sphere. To maintain the spherical shape of the globe, the eyeball must be pressurised from within by fluid, and this pressure is contained by a strong outer coat – the white sclera (Gr=hard). This coat withstands trauma and infection well, so these problems are generally confined to the surrounding tissues outside the eyeball and only occasionally is the eye itself infected.

In order to admit light, the front of the sclera, the cornea, must be completely transparent, which means that it is devoid of capillaries for the provision of nourishment. This must therefore be provided by the tears from the lacrimal glands and by the aqueous humour in the anterior chamber, and damage to either mechanism results in lack of translucency. Moreover the corner must be well protected, a function of the very sensitive membrane, the conjunctiva, which covers it, and also the lids which close reflexly in the event of threat. Finally, because the light reflected from an object is divergent, it must be concentrated on the light sensitive area, the retina, by a focussing mechanism, the lens, or we would see the world through a keyhole. Of course the lens inverts the image on the screen, so we actually see the world upside down and leave it to our occipital cortex to right it again.

In such an immensely complex apparatus it is surprising that so few elements fail us, apart from the focussing mechanism for which we may need help. The most commonly occurring faults are in the lids and lacrimal apparatus, sometimes in the conjunctival membrane and less

211

often on the cornea. Within the eyeball, apart from refractive errors, the usual problem is with ageing changes in the lens – cataract, disorders of pressurisation – glaucoma and least often retinal and neural problems. Finally it must be remembered that the eyes operate as a pair and each looks at an object from a slightly different angle. Failure to do this results in a squint (strabismus), most frequently seen in children.

LACRIMAL PROBLEMS

These are often seen in the period shortly after birth, in babies suffering from *sticky eye* which is caused by a narrowing of the tear duct where it crosses the orbital bone just below the eye. Quite often the duct is immature and does not fully develop for several months, during which time the tears well up and overflow down the cheeks. During the night they form a stagnant pool which evaporates and thickens, so that on waking the eyelids are encrusted and stuck together, some-times slightly infected. Treatment is to bathe away the crusts and then gently massage the lacrimal duct just below the inner corner of the eye. It is rare for the duct to need probing or syringing unless it fails to resolve spontaneously in 3–4 months. On occasions a similar condition may occur in adults, and lead to the symptom of *epiphora* – tears running down the cheeks.

Another cause of epiphora, usually in the elderly, is failure of the entrance of the lacrimal duct to approximate to the eyeball, because the tissues of the lower lid have either atrophied or been displaced by a Meibomiam cyst (qv), giving the eye a red-rimmed appearance. This turning out of the lid is known as an *ectropion*, and the opposite condition or *entropion* leads to a similar result by allowing the lashes to abrade the conjunctiva.

In the hollow just below the inner aspect of the eye lies the lacrimal sac, a reservoir of tears which may sometimes be the focus for infection. A swollen, inflamed cyst appears, known as a 'dacryocystitis' (Gr. dacryos= tear), which on pressure will yield some pus oozing out of the punctum on the lower lid, and the eye will water.

Sjogren's syndrome is a condition of atrophy of the lacrimal glands, and this causes gradual loss of their secretions, leading to itching, grittiness and recurrent inflammation of the conjunctiva. It usually starts in middle-age, especially in women around the time of the menopause, and may be associated with rheumatoid arthritis or other connective tissue disorders. There is sometimes accompanying dryness of the salivary glands with dry mouth and soreness of the tongue.

THE LIDS

These are covered in front by a relatively thin layer of skin and so are prone to a number of skin conditions, especially allergies and eczema, while behind the lid is the conjunctival membrane which becomes inflamed in conjunctivitis (qv). At its centre the lid is stiffened by a plate of connective tissue – the tarsus, and it is here that tarsal cysts may arise from small glands within the tarsus known as Meibomian glands, whose function is to secrete sebaceous fluid which lubricates the lids.

Meibomian or *tarsal cysts* are not true cysts caused by blockage of a duct, but enlargement of the glandular tissue due to chronic irritation or infection, and they tend to occur in crops. The gland becomes swollen and red, when it is known as a 'chalazion' (Gr. = a collection of rubble), being particularly prominent if the lid is everted and the back inspected, so the patient may complain of watering and irritation. Sometimes they become acutely inflamed and discharge pus, but can be differentiated from a stye (see below) by the position half way up the lid.

A *stye* or 'hordeolum' (L. hordeum = barley) is an infection of the root of a lash, and thus is always found at the edge of the lid where it causes an inflamed swelling with a yellow head. Styes often contain staphylococci and there may be similar skin infections about such as boils.

Blepharitis (Gr. blepharon – eyelid) is a chronic inflammation of the margin of the lids which become red, scaly and sometimes slightly swollen or even ulcerating. This condition is found in those predisposed to dandruff or seborrhoea, and tends to lead to recurrent infections, including styes. The greasy scales cling to the lashes and may be removed by bathing with 5% bicarbonate of soda in warm water. On occasions a more widespread blepharitis is a result of an allergy to cosmetics or eye drops.

Ptosis (Gr. = falling) is the term given to drooping of the upper lid from paralysis of the muscles, most cases being congenital. In old age so-called 'senile ptosis' is simply due to sagging of the tissues which have become atrophied. Ptosis of sudden onset is more significant and if unilateral is then due either to paralysis of the third cranial nerve or to the sympathetic nerves in the neck (usually from a bronchial carcinoma). The latter leads to the triad of symptoms known as *Horner's syndrome*, a combination of ptosis, a sunken eye and a constricted pupil. Of course if the sympathetic nerves are stimulated the lids will do the opposite and rotract, and this is what helps to cause the staring eyes seen in hyperthyroidism.

Myaesthenia gravis is a disease characterised by a general weakness of the muscles, and is a classical autoimmune disease in which the supplies of the neurotransmitter acetylcholine conducting the nerve impulse across the neuromuscular junction becomes depleted. All the muscles are affected to some degree, but the most prominent feature is usually bilateral ptosis, and the lids drop progressively as the day wears on, followed by weakness of the other muscles of the body.

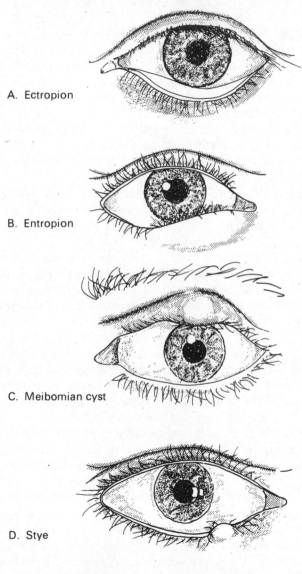

A. Ectropion

B. Entropion

C. Meibomian cyst

D. Stye

FIGURE 19.1   *Disorders of the eyelids*

A skin condition which has a preference for the eyelids is *xanthelasma* (Gr. xanthos = yellow; elasma = plate) – thickened, yellow, waxy plaques on the upper or lower lids near the inner canthus. These plaques signify excessive quantities of cholesterol in the blood, and so are seen in those with familial *hypercholesterolaemia*, an inherited condition, and also in some diabetics.

THE CONJUNCTIVA

This is the membrane which lines the back of the lids and also covers the front of the eyeball, so that when the eyes are closed it forms a complete sac containing tears. Not infrequently it becomes inflamed owing to exposure to dust, infection and allergens such as pollen, giving rise to various types of conjunctivitis. A very frequently met condition of the conjunctiva is a *subconjunctival haemorrhage*, which follows a spontaneous rupture of one of the capillaries and spreads a layer of blood across the white sclera, disfiguring the eye for a week or two but of no pathological significance.

Acute conjunctivitis is commonly due to bacterial infection, and if it is restricted to one eye this indicates that a foreign body is the probable cause. The sclera of the eye is pink or red and swollen, especially at the periphery, as is the tarsal conjunctiva, and epiphora may be prominent. Sometimes there is much oedema, a condition known as 'chemosis', and there may be a purulent discharge which sticks the lids together, along with some flecks of mucopus seen under the lids. The vision is essentially normal and the pupil is a regular shape and reacts to light.

If the condition occurs in a newborn baby then a gonorrhoeal cause must be considered – so-called 'ophthalmia neonatorum' – as this is a virulent infection which may lead to blindness if inadequately treated. It is, however, rare nowadays and most cases of neonatal conjunctivitis are associated with a chlamydial infection and called 'inclusion conjunctivitis' because of the way the chlamydia are included within the cells. The mother will usually be found to have a venereal infection. This form is occasionally caught by adults in swimming baths and seems to be becoming more common.

Trachoma is also a chlamydial conjunctivitis, rare in this country but on a world wide scale it is the most common cause of blindness. Cases are occasionally seen among immigrants from the middle and far east, appearing as chronic conjunctivitis.

Viral conjunctivitis occurs in schools and other communities as a local outbreak of 'pink eye', with slight fever and enlargement of the pre-auricular glands in front of the ear. There is a pink tinge to the sclera, and the eye waters considerably, but it lasts only a few days and usually clears spontaneously.

Allergic conjunctivitis is not as a rule difficult to distinguish from an infective cause, and produces a clear, watery discharge with much itching. It assumes two forms, the first being that of hay fever and occurring in the summer months in conjunction with sneezing and catarrh. Less commonly a different, more localised allergy involving just the tarsal conjunctiva may occur, known as *vernal* or *spring catarrh* as it appears earlier in the year. The back of the lids assume a very swollen and rather alarming 'cobblestone' appearance, with large itchy swellings and characteristic ropy secretions.

A *pterygium* (GR. = wing) is sometimes seen on the nasal side of the eyeball, crossing the sclera as an opaque triangular encroachment. It is a degenerative change in the conjunctiva and mostly seen in dry, sunny countries where UV light is thought to be a causative factor. Unless it grows large enough to invade the cornea it is only really of cosmetic significance and has no effect on vision.

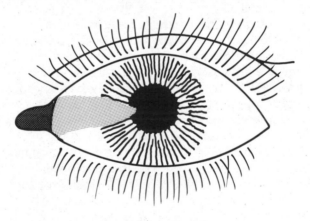

FIGURE 19.2A   *Pterygium*

THE CORNEA

The most frequently seen lesion on the cornea is the crescent or circle of lipid material, thickest at the top or bottom, termed an *arcus senilis*. It is separated from the margin of the cornea by a thin band of clear cornea and is a greyish colour. When seen in younger people it usually signifies an abnormally large quantity of lipid in the blood and is therefore associated with vascular pathology, but it never extends far enough toward the centre to affect sight.

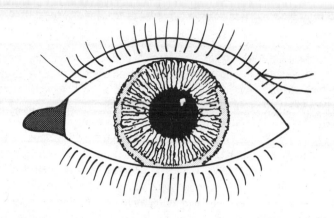

FIGURE 19.2B   *Arcus senilis*

Inflammation of the cornea is termed *keratitis* and is usually associated with viruses as, with the exception of the gonococcus, bacteria can only invade the corneal epithelium if it is already damaged. It is for this reason that a corneal abrasion needs regular scrutiny to ensure that it does not become a corneal ulcer. The cornea is also damaged by drying as may

TABLE 19.1	Possible causes of a painful eye
Condition	**Pointers**
Conjunctivitis	Red, watery conjunctiva, usually bilateral
Foreign body	Sudden onset, spasm of lid
Stye	Visible at root of lash
Blepharitis	Rash on lid, may be from contact
Entropion	Lid turned inward, watering
Meibomian cyst	Only if infected
Sinusitis	Over or under eye, tender to press
Dendritic ulcer	Severe pain, visual impairment, difficult to spot
Glaucoma	Halos around lights, visual disturbance, oval pupil
Iritis	Central pattern of erythema, visual disturbance
Dacryocystitis	Inflammation under eye, swelling
Temporal arteritis	Age, general symptoms, tender artery
Acne rosacea	Mild discomfort, espiscleritis, facial rash
Optic neuritis	Deep discomfort, worse on moving eye especially upwards

occur in Sjogren's syndrome, trachoma and the exophthalmos of thyrotoxicosis if the lids fail to meet. Acne rosacea may lead to keratitis in some, and will improve as the skin condition resolves.

Herpes simplex keratitis is a form of cold sore occurring on the cornea, and takes the shape of tiny pinhead size dots or a ragged, branching ulcer known from its shape as *dendritic* (Gr. dendron = tree). Needless to say the condition is extremely painful, with photophobia and reddening of the sclera, along with some impairment of vision. Herpes zoster or *shingles* may also occur on the cornea if the ophthalmic nerve is affected and a blistering rash is seen on the forehead and down the side of the nose. This mostly affects elderly patients and is preceded and sometimes followed by a neuralgic pain along the course of the nerve, which may be very severe and persistent. With both forms of keratitis, if a deep ulcer forms in the cornea then there is inflammation of the anterior chamber and the iris. Pus may gravitate to form a level at the bottom of the anterior chamber – a 'hypopyon', and the iris then becomes swollen and engorged with blood – *acute iritis* (also sometimes called iridocyclitis).

THE UVEAL TRACT

Fig 19.4 illustrates the proximity of the iris, ciliary body and choroid which are continuous with one another and together termed the 'uvea' or 'uveal tract' (Gr. uvea = hump-backed), and inflammation of the area is often termed *uveitis*. This has come to be virtually synonymous for 'iritis', 'iridocyclitis' and 'choroiditis' and the three expressions may be regarded as interchangeable.

Since the uvea is enclosed within the eyeball, most cases of uveitis are not of infective origin but have an allergic or autoimmune basis. It seems that the cells of the iris are extremely sensitive to antigens and if one appears in the blood, as may happen in the chronic conditions mentioned below, the tissue reacts by inflaming and swelling, so uveitis is characterised by a deep, throbbing pain in the eye, quite unlike the sharp pains of keratitis. There is some redness to be seen but this is just at the edge of the cornea as a rule and does not involve the whole conjunctival sac. There is also marked constriction of the pupil, which is unfortunate as the congested iris is likely to become stuck to the lens immediately behind it by the exudate, and remain an irregular shape on account of these adhesions or 'synechiae' as they are termed (Gr. synechio = dance together). This is the reason for using atropine drops to dilate the pupil and prevent these adhesions occurring.

The conditions mainly associated with uveitis are rheumatoid arthritis, sarcoidosis, ankylosing spondylitis, Reiter's syndrome, lupus

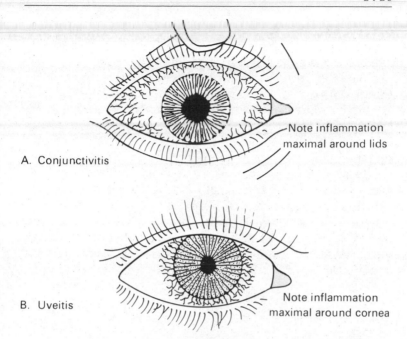

A. Conjunctivitis

Note inflammation
maximal around lids

B. Uveitis

Note inflammation
maximal around cornea

C. Dendritic ulcer

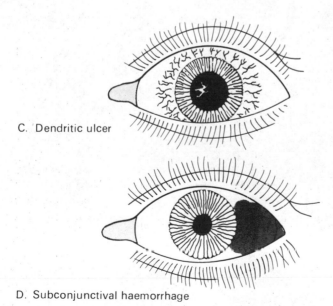

D. Subconjunctival haemorrhage

FIGURE 19.3   *The common causes of a red eye*

erythematosis and Behcet's disease. The latter is an uncommon but very distressing and painful condition of unknown origin occurring mostly in young men who, as well as the iritis, develop ulceration of the mouth and genitalia.

GLAUCOMA

The pressure within the eye has to be finely balanced so that it is sufficient to maintain the roundness of the eyeball but not so great that it prevents blood from entering to nourish the retina. If it exceeds what is considered normal, about 20 mmHg as measured on the tonometer, then the retina will become ischaemic and there ensues the condition known as glaucoma. This develops because the outflow of the aqueous humour in the anterior chamber is obstructed, sometimes because the shape of the eye allows the lens to push the iris forward (*closed angle* or *acute glaucoma*), but often for no obvious reason (open angle or *chronic glaucoma*). In a few cases it may be secondary to uveitis which silts up the drainage channel with inflammatory debris.

Canal where aqueous is absorbed   Canal obstructed

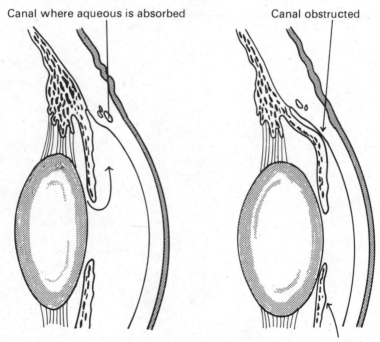

Iris pushed forward by large myopic lens

FIGURE 19.4   *The circulation of aqueous humour in A. normal eye and B. acute glaucoma*

Acute glaucoma occurs particularly in women in their 50s and 60s, and is due to narrowing of the angle of the anterior chamber by a large lense in a relatively small eye, so the patient is usually longsighted and wears thick glasses. Attacks come on suddenly after the pupil has dilated and closed the angle altogether, often at night, and are characterised by blurred vision, headaches and the appearance of coloured haloes around lights (Gr. glaucos=gleaming). These attacks recur and become more severe until there is intense congestion of the eye and serious visual damage. The orthodox treatment involves removing a small piece of the iris in each eye (peripheral iridectomy), to allow the humour to pass directly into the drainage channel.

Chronic glaucoma, also known as simple glaucoma, is more insidious in its manner of approach, and arises mostly in elderly people. It appears in eyes of all shapes and sizes and the exact cause is unknown. There may be a few slight headaches but in most patients the only evidence is the gradual loss of the outer part of the field of vision, known as a *scotoma*, and this may pass unnoticed for many weeks. It is because of this that regular examination of the eye and measurement of the pressure by an optician is desirable in this age group. If the retina is examined with an ophthalmoscope, a characteristic cup-shaped depression in the optic disc can be seen where the retina sags at its weakest point. Standard treatment is with pilocarpine or adrenaline drops to encourage the outflow, or beta-blocking drops to reduce the production of humour.

CATARACT

The name derives from the Greek meaning 'accursed', and illustrates the dread in which patients hold this opacity of the lens, heralding as it does the last of the seven ages of man (and woman, for it occurs equally in both sexes). The age at which so-called 'senile cataract' starts is determined by genetic influence, as is the speed with which it progresses.

Cataracts are caused by the coagulation of the proteins of the lens with age, much as egg albumen coagulates on heating, and the opacities begin as wedge-shaped spokes around the edge of the lens with clear areas in between. These actually begin in early middle age, but we are not aware of them as that part of the lens is covered by the iris, and visual acuity is maximum through the centre of the lens. Eventually these wedges converge on the hub and obscure central vision, creating the need for large print books which no spectacles can assist. As well as spreading centrally, the opacities spread from the inner layers of the lens to the outer (the lens is made of layers rather like an onion), and until they have reached the cortex the cataract is not 'complete' and therefore technically more difficult to extract. Once it has become ripe it then starts to disintegrate and cause complications, so there is an optimal time at which to remove it, and this is not always understood by patients who feel that their vision will be dramatically restored at the sweep of a scalpel. Recently the tendency has been to insert a small plastic lens in place of the natural one, and use spectacles to change the focal length when required. Sometimes this is not feasible and a contact lens of thick spectacles are used instead, but this has the disadvantage of magnifying everything and distorting vision.

The process of hydration and coagulation which leads to cataracts may be accelerated in certain circumstances, and *diabetes*, long-term *steroid therapy*, infra-red light and trauma are all liable to cause early cataracts. Congenital cataracts can occur in rubella and Down's syndrome.

RETINAL DISORDERS

The retina, like any other tissue, may suffer from a variety of pathology – oedema, ischaemia, degeneration, detachment and even infection. However, because of its central role as a sensory receptor, it responds by informing us immediately and at the least provocation.

Interference with the blood supply to the retina may arise particularly in *diabetes* and *hypertension*, and leads to both leakage from the vessels at the back of the 'fundus' of the eye, and to oedema of the retina (*papilloedema*), although this is only visible with an opthalmoscope. Blindness in this country most commonly results from so-called *diabetic retinopathy* which is a mixture of lack of nourishment, haemorrhage and exudation of fat, especially around the macula where central vision is located and damage is therefore maximal. Furthermore, the ischaemic retina responds by prompting the growth of new vessels out into the vitreous humour which only makes matters worse, and it is for the destruction of these that diabetics undergo laser treatment.

Senile macular degeneration is the name given to the atrophy of cells in the macula of the retina which sometimes takes place in the elderly and leads to a central scotoma affecting the reading area of the eye. A slightly similar condition, though with a totally different cause and affecting a much younger age group is *retinitis pigmentosa*, an inherited tendency to degeneration and pigmentation of the cones and even more the rods. This starts in childhood as night-blindness and leads to gradual tunnel vision and then complete blindness in middle age as the degeneration encroaches on the macula.

Retinal detachment is actually a split in the two layers of the retina, either due to a tear in the retina allowing vitreous fluid to seep through and raise the inner layer off its bed, as is seen in diabetes or a sudden blow to the eye; or else because the inner layer becomes attached to the vitreous which tugs at it and produces the standard retinal response – flashing lights. These are a warning that a detachment is impending, and can be differentiated from those of migraine by always being in exactly the same place. Once a detachment occurs, there is no pain but a curtain begins to fall across the field of vision as the retina comes away, and needs to be gently replaced and probably affixed with the judicious use of a coagulating laser.

Floaters or 'muscae volitantes' (L. musca = fly; volito = fluttering) are a different phenomenon altogether and consist of particles of collagen and other debris floating in the vitreous and observable by the subject against a light background and by the practitioner with an ophthalmoscope. Unless they suddenly appear in large numbers they are not pathological, but need to be carefully distinguished from the flashing lights of impending detachment mentioned above.

SQUINT

In normal development a newborn baby learns to focus its eyes on an object within a few weeks, and to do so it must have attained macular vision. During the learning process the eyes wander independently of one another, but soon learn that by working simultaneously as a pair they are able to judge the distance of an object, so binocular vision arrives. But what happens if one eye has greater difficulty in seeing than the other, either from a refractive error in the lens or from more serious pathology? This eye will then have difficulty focussing on the object, and even if it does the image will be in the wrong place and so double vision occurs which simply confuses the child. So the brain automatically suppresses the false image and the eye in question becomes lazy or *amblyopic* (Gr. amblyos = dim) and gradually ceases to function at all. Over the next few years the suppression continues until by the age of five or so it is permanent and the child is left with monocular vision. Moreover the amblyopic eye feels under no compunction to follow its colleague in the direction of its gaze and remains a social embarrassment to its owner who finds as he gets older that the wrong people (who he can't see) keep answering his questions.

Until the amblyopic eye finally gives up, the child may look at objects with either eye 'alternate fixation' – but will not, as is sometimes believed, 'grow out of a squint'. In order to encourage the weaker eye to develop macular vision it is necessary to cover the good eye with a patch or even, if the image is falling far outside the macula, to correct the eye muscles surgically.

Sudden squints arising in adults may be due to damage to one of the nerves supplying the extrinsic eye muscles, usually from diabetes, MS or occasionally a tumour or aneurysm compressing the nerve. These will cause diplopia for a few days until the false image is suppressed. Equally a squint can occur if there is loss of vision in one eye as the eye will then have no object to fix on and keep it steady.

CHAPTER TWENTY

EAR:
DISORDERS OF
HEARING & BALANCE

*T*he ear is the organ of both hearing and balance, two of our most important senses, and is well protected by being sited deep within the temporal bone. This means that only the external canal and the ear drum are easily examined, and the functions of the middle and inner ear must be inferred from special tests. Examination of the drum is by using an otoscope (auroscope), and will be made easier if the canal is straightened by gently pulling the ear upwards and backwards.

THE EXTERNAL EAR

The pinna or auricle is a rudimentary funnel for sound which has little use in humans, and consists simply of cartilage covered in skin, although a few people retain the vestigial muscles which enable it to be moved. The crease behind the auricle is the site of numerous sebaceous glands which secrete a greasy substance, and is a common site for sebaceous cysts to form. The helix, which is the upper part of the pinna, occasionally contains a tophus in gouty subjects, or is disfigured from repeated bruising in boxers with 'cauliflower ears'. The outer part of the external auditory canal contains glands which secrete a similar oily substance which solidifies with time to form wax, the colour depending on its age and water content. Some individuals make more wax than others, and it is notable that the contraceptive pill reduces the amount of wax secretion. Wax has a protective quality and ensures that water is repelled, as well as killing bacteria by its acidic nature, and people with insufficient wax are liable to suffer from repeated attacks of infection of the canal.

Many of the problems of the external auditory canal are those of the skin which line it, and as this is a warm, moist locality eczema commonly features here and causes a chronic, itchy discharge and sometimes some small blisters. It may periodically become infected, especially if abraded by instruments used for cleaning wax from the ear, and then becomes painful, extremely so if a boil is present and will then be seen blocking the canal. *Otitis externa* is particularly likely to occur after swimming in dirty water when fungi can enter and set up a cheesy, white discharge, and if the subject is a child the possibility of a foreign body must be remembered as this is a favourite site for depositing small objects.

THE DRUM

The drum or *tympanic membrane* is an oval, semi-transparent membrane the size of a large pea in diameter, and set at the end of the 1" long canal. It is normally a delicate pearly grey colour, and when inflamed goes angry red and later a deep purple. This will happen if a middle ear infection occurs, or after swimming and diving or flying in pressurised aircraft, on account of the imbalance between the pressures on the different sides of the drum, known as *barotrauma*. During flight the aircraft is normally pressurised at a rather lower than normal pressure and some air leaves the Eustachian tube. On touchdown the pressure is then brought to normal but if the air is unable to re-enter the tube because of catarrh then the drum will bulge inwards and severe pain may result along with deafness and vertigo, lasting several hours.

Perforations of the drum are almost always the result of middle ear infections (see below), and if they occur in the lower part of the membrane and are not too large then they will usually heal uneventfully within a short time. For the duration they will discharge a thin water pus, but because they seldom lead to complications they are sometimes termed 'safe' perforations. A few people develop a large hole, sometimes as a result of blast damage, and this may require a graft before it will heal.

If the perforation is in the upper part of the tympanic membrane it is termed an 'unsafe perforation', because such lesions will tend to become chronic and gradually erode the underlying bone structures, particularly the ossicles and the mastoid bone. Over a long period of time the infection builds up into a mass of granulomatous tissue termed a *cholesteatoma* which exudes a profuse and offensive discharge. This is liable to create abscesses and infections within the temporal bone and result in surgery, so such a perforation must be treated with great circumspection.

THE MIDDLE EAR

Otitis media is one of the commonest of childhood complaints and tends to occur whenever there is blockage of the Eustachian tube at the lower end on account of catarrh or enlarged adenoids. If a cold or other upper respiratory infection occurs then it will often progress upward into the middle ear and cause pain of a stabbing or throbbing nature. The secretions will become infected with staphylococci or streptococci and the drum will be seen to bulge under pressure from the pus and possibly eventually burst, which relieves the pain. If the drum does not perforate it will still heal fairly quickly within a week or so, and develop a scaly appearance for a while, rather like crazy paving.

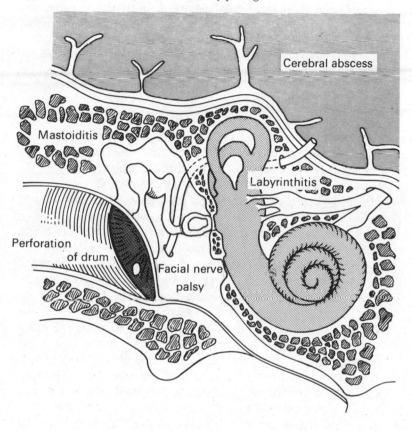

FIGURE 20.1   *The complications of otitis media*

Complications of otitis media usually involve extensions of the infection into neighbouring areas, and although uncommon they need to be kept in mind as they are potentially serious.

    – *Mastoiditis* is one of the better known and occurs when infection travels into the hollow spaces of the mastoid bone behind the ear, which may happen quite suddenly. The bone becomes tender when pressed (and this should always be tested), there is swelling there and the auricle is pushed forward and protrudes more than its opposite when seen from the front. If a course of antibiotics given for the ear infections has been aborted then mastoiditis may be masked and build up slowly with increasing pain in the ear.

– Extension of the infection upwards can very rarely penetrate the temporal bone and invade the meninges to cause *meningitis* or a *cerebral abscess*, when the patient will suddenly become severely ill and comatose.

– The facial nerve runs across the Eustachian tube and so it is liable to damage here in the form of *Bell's palsy* (see chapter 18).

– The inner ear may become involved which will announce itself by the vertigo and vomiting of *labyrinthitis*.

Glue ears is a familiar condition which is being diagnosed more and more frequently, and one child in 200 is now operated on every year for the insertion of grommets. Because the Eustachian tube is kept full of air at atmospheric presure by opening the lower end each time we swallow, the ear ossicles are able to vibrate unimpeded. If, however, the tube becomes full of fluid then gradually the hearing is impaired and speech and language development is lost at a critical age.

The middle ear, being lined by mucus membrane, normally secretes a small amount of mucus and if this cannot drain it gradually thickens until it takes on the colour and consistency of glue. Because the lower end of the tube is so easily impeded by enlarged adenoids, a negative pressure builds up in the middle ear which sucks mucus out of the glands. At one time the adenoids were removed in the hope that this would relieve the situation, but it is now found to be less traumatic to simply relieve the vacuum at the other end by inserting small tubes in the drum called *grommets*, so that air can enter and allow the ossicles to vibrate freely. These tiny grommets, about the size of a split pea, usually stay in place for about six months before being spontaneously rejected. In about one child in five the grommets will need to be reinserted, and during the time of having them in place they should wear ear plugs when swimming and not dive beneath the water.

Otosclerosis is a genetic disorder of the ossicles of the middle ear, especially the last in the chain, the stapes. The bone first becomes spongy and then hardens ('sclerosis') and cements itself to the oval window beyond, so that vibrations are impeded, especially those of a higher frequency. Another consequence is that the stapedius reflex initially over-reacts, and as the function of this tiny muscle is to act as a 'damper' for loud noise, these are excluded and so speech is heard better against a background of noise ('paracusis').

The hearing loss which ensues is usually bilateral and is first noticed by young adults in their 20s and 30s, becoming progressively worse into middle-age at which point it may require treatment with more than just a hearing aid. In women the deafness may suddenly worsen during pregnancy or if they go on the Pill, and as both sexes may experience a little vertigo the condition may be misinterpreted as Meniere's disease. The orthodox treatment involves removal of the stapes and its replacement with a small plastic piston, and this generates substantial improvement in the majority of sufferers. There is also some evidence that small doses of fluoride and calcium stabilises the bone and helps to halt the deterioration.

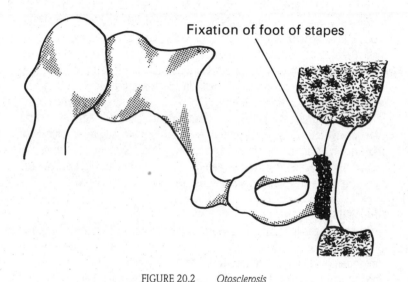

Fixation of foot of stapes

FIGURE 20.2   *Otosclerosis*

THE INNER EAR

Because the cochlea and the vestibular labyrinth lie so close together and share the vestibulochlear nerve, the symptom of deafness or tinnitus is often accompanied by vertigo. This is particularly seen in *Meniere's disease*, where there is a sudden increase in the pressure within the labyrinth for reasons which are not clear. The result is that periodically there is distortion of the labyrinth and episodes of vertigo and nausea, tinnitus and fluctuation hearing loss along with a sense of pressure in the ears. The attacks vary in frequency from one every few months to one a week and may build up over the years, but in between attacks the patient is relatively symptom free.

An individual attack will often come on very suddenly and last from a few hours to several days, effectively confining the patient to bed from the vertigo. As well as these symptoms some sufferers also notice increasing deafness over the years in between the acute attacks, especially for the lower notes, and also a degree of tinnitus. For some reason the fair-skinned, blue-eyed types seem to develop Meniere's disease more readily, usually between the ages of 30–60.

VERTIGO

This whirling sensation, often described as giddiness or dizziness, is not an uncommon symptom of other disorders but may occur on its own. *Benign positional vertigo* is the name given to that which occurs only when the head is in a certain position, such as when shaving, seemingly because certain hair cells in the ampulla are easily stimulated. Elderly people are particularly liable to this, but it is usually fatigueable, i.e. it passes off in a few minutes if they maintain the head in that position and then they will be symptom free for several hours.

Labyrinthitis is an occasional consequence of a cold or other viral infection when the labyrinth becomes inflamed and begins to pass false information resulting in severe vertigo which is worse on moving the head. This may lead to extreme nausea and vomiting and last for several days or more, but always clears without serious consequences.

DEAFNESS

Loss of hearing is in many ways more tragic than loss of sight, for whereas the blind are isolated from things, the deaf are isolated from people and consequently become very lonely. There is a tendency for our organ of Corti to deteriorate with the years, and it is the peripheral cells, the ones which sense the higher notes, which go first. This *presbyacusis*, as the deafness of age is termed (L. presbus=old), is also contributed to by an increasing stiffness of the drum which lowers the amplitude of sound generally.

Generally speaking there are two types of deafness, those which arise in the chain of conduction through the outer and middle ear, *conduction deafness*, and those whose origins are in the cochlea, cochlear nerve or even in the brain *perceptive deafness* or *sensorineural deafness*. The latter is very much less amenable to treatment owing to its pathology, whereas conductive deafness can at least be helped by a hearing aid if nothing else, as this will amplify sound through the temporal bone itself.

Wax is the commonest reason for conductive deafness, formed by the specialised ceruminous glands in the skin to protect the canal from dirt and water, and which normally clears itself. Some people make large quantities of wax and their ears may require regular syringing. We have already mentioned such things as otitis media, glue ears and otosclerosis as causes of either muffled hearing or deafness. If one ear is blocked from conducting sound the body is unable to locate the origin of a noise as it relies on the minute difference in timing of the arrival of the sound in the two ears in order to pinpoint the source.

Perceptive deafness is most commonly a result of acoustic trauma, especially in the higher frequencies such as are encountered in many rock bands and in industry. The deterioration is gradual but relentless, and measurement of hearing with audiometry will give an early warning of trouble by indicating the typical dip in high frequency response at around 4 kHz. To some extent the degree of deafness depends on the duration of exposure to noise combined with the time allowed for recovery, and continuous noise, such as is encountered in some work situations, is especially hazardous. The louder the noise, the longer time is required to recover, and those who fought on the dreadnoughts of old spent many days after a battle unable to hear even the sound of their own voice.

TINNITUS

Deafness and tinnitus may go hand in hand, tinnitus being the reaction of the organ of Corti in the cochlea to some kind of stimulus such as inflammation or pressure, while perceptive deafness is the failure to react to that stimulus. Tinnitus is a common and often very distressing disorder, experienced as a continual noise in the head and ranging from a high pitched whistle to a deep booming vibration. Occasionally it is the result of the rushing of blood through the arteries around the temporal area, and can be brought about by high blood pressure or anaemia, but the great majority of cases, of which there are about 100,000 in the UK, arise for no obvious reason.

It has been recognised that certain drugs, especially antibiotics such as streptomycin, can lead to both tinnitus and deafness, and that aspirin and quinine both cause ringing in the ears. Tinnitus may arise after a head injury, as a result of exposure to excessive noise, after lead poisoning or as one of the symptoms of Meniere's disease or otosclerosis. Arteriosclerosis of the artery supplying the cochlea is thought to cause deterioration of the organ leading to tinnitus in some. There is also a theory that tinnitus results from the minute currents set up in the region by mercury fillings in the teeth, and some have found relief by having their fillings removed.

Paradoxically a hearing aid may help control the symptoms by allowing more sound to stimulate the cochlea which pushes the tinnitus into the background. In a similar vein a masker can be used to generate sound of the same pitch as the tinnitus and this may even suppress the noise completely for a few hours so it is most useful in the evening before going to bed to ensure a good night's sleep.

GLOSSARY OF MEDICAL & HOMOEOPATHIC TERMS

(Words followed by an asterisk indicate that they are no longer in common usage).

ABSCESS – A local collection of pus
ACHALASIA – Inability of organ to relax
ACHLORHYDRIA – Absence of acid in the stomach
ACIDOSIS – Excess acidity of the blood
ADENITIS – Inflammation of a gland
ADENOMA – Benign tumour of glandular tissue
-aemia – Pertaining to the blood
AETIOLOGY – The cause of a disease
AGUE* – Intermittent fever
ALBUMINURIA – Presence of albumen in the urine
AMAUROSIS – Transient blindness
AMBLYOPIA – Dimness of vision
AMENORRHOEA – Absence of periods
ANALGESIA – Without pain
ANAPHYLAXIS – Generalised severe allergic reaction
ANASARCA* – Generalised oedema
Angio- – Pertaining to the blood vessels
ANKYLOSIS – Bony fusion
ANOREXIA – Without appetite
ANOXIA – Deficiency of oxygen in the blood
ANTIBODY – Specific substance produced by body in response to antigen
ANTIGEN – Substance which the body recognises as not itself
ANURIA – Not passing urine
APHASIA – Inability to formulate words in the brain
APHONIA – Inability to convert thoughts into speech
APHTHOUS – Painful and ulcerated (usually mouth)
ARRHYTHMIA – Abnormal cardiac rhythm
ARTHRALGIA – Painful joints, not necessarily swollen
ARTHROPATHY – Joint disease, not necessarily painful
ASCITES – Oedema fluid in the peritoneal cavity
ASTHENIA* – Generalised weakness

ATAXIA – Unbalanced, staggering
ATOPY – Form of hypersensitivity
ATROPHY – Withering, loss of size and function
ATTENUATED – Rendered less harmful

BACTERIURIA – Presence of bacteria in urine
BALANITIS – Inflammation of glans penis
BALANOPOSTHITIS – Same as balanitis, but including foreskin
BENIGN – Innocent, non life-threatening
BLEPHARITIS – Inflammation of eyelid
BORBORYGMI – Noises made by peristalsis
BRADYCARDIA – Slow heart beat
BRUIT – Noise made by blood in narrowed or tortuous vessel
BUBO* – Syphilitic gland in the groin
BUCCAL – Mucus membrane of inside of cheek
BULIMIA – Pathologically excessive appetite
BULLA – A large blister

CACHEXIA – Emaciation
CALCULUS – Stone
CARCINOGEN – Cancer-producing substance
CASTS – Exucates from kidney tubules seen in urine
CATAMENIA* – Periods
CELLULITIS – Inflammation of connective tissue
CHALAZION – Inflamed Meibomian cyst on eyelid
CHEMOSIS – Oedema of conjunctival membrane
CHLOROSIS* – Iron deficiency of puberty
CHORDEE* – Painful involuntary erection seen in gonorrhoea
CHOREA – Involuntary writhing movements
CICATRIX* – Scar
CLIMACTERIC – The changes accompanying the menopause
CLONUS/CLONIC – Alternating contraction and relaxation of a
                             muscle
COARCTATION – Narrowing
CONDYLOMATA – Venereal warts
CONTAGIOUS – Transmitted by touch
CORTEX – Outer part or layer of an organ
CREPITATION – Crackling sound
CYANOSIS – Blue discolouration of blood from increase in CO_2
CYST – A sac enclosing fluid
-cyte – Type of cell

DACRYOCYSTITIS Inflammation of tear gland
DEMENTIA – Deterioration of mental faculties
DERMOGRAPHIA – Visible reaction of skin to touch or pressure
DIALYSIS – Separation of substance through a porous membrane
DIAPHORESIS* – Increased perspiration
DIASTOLE – Relaxation phase of the heart
DIATHESIS* – Constitutional predisposition
DIPLOPIA – Double vision
DIURESIS – Passing increased quantity of urine
DROPSY* – Generalised oedema
Dys – Under or malfunction in some way
DYSARTHRIA – Difficulty speaking words
DYSLEXIA – Difficulty reading
DYSMENORRHOEA – Painful periods
DYSPEPSIA – Painful digestion
DYSPHASIA – Difficulty assembling speech in brain
DYSPNOEA – Shortness of breath
DYSTROPHY – Defective development
DYSURIA – Painful urination

ECCHYMOSIS – Large bruise
ECLAMPSIA – Fit associated with pregnancy
ECTHEMA – Local area of infection of skin which heals with scarring
-ectomy – Removal by surgery
EFFUSION – Extravasation of fluid into cavity
EMBOLISM – Obstruction of blood vessel by any form of wedge
EMETIC – Substance which induces vomiting
EMPHYSEMA – Distension of tissues, usually lung
EMPYEMA – Collection of pus in a hollow organ
ENDOTHELIUM – Internal lining
ENURESIS – Urinating in the bed
EPISTAXIS – Nosebleed
EPITHELIUM – External covering
ERUCTATION – Belching
ERYTHEMA – Reddening
ERYTHISM* – Overexcitability
E.S.R. – Erythrocyte sedimentation rate

FEBRICULA* – Short, mild fever
FELON – Inflammation of side of nail
FIBRILLATION – Irregular heart beat caused by overexcitable myocardium

235

FIBROMA – Benign tumour of fibrous tissue
FIBROSIS – The formation of fibrous tissue
FISTULA – Pathological connection between two epithelial surfaces
FLATUS – Gas in the intestines
FOETOR – Offensive odour
FORMICATION* – Sensation as if ants were crawling over the skin
FURUNCLE – Boil

GANGLION – Collection of nerve cells outside the CNS/cyst of a joint
GANGRENE – Death of tissue, usually from inadequate blood supply
GINGIVITIS – Inflammation of gums
GLEET* – Mucoid discharge from the penis
GLOSSAL – Pertaining to the tongue
GLYCOGEN – Form in which carbohydrate is stored in liver and muscles
GOITRE – Thyroid swelling
GRANULOMA – Clusters of cells in chronic inflammation
GUMMA – Swelling seen in tertiary syphilis

HAEMATEMESIS – Vomiting blood
HAEMATURIA – Passing blood in the urine
HAEMOLYSIS – Breakdown of erythrocytes liberating haemoglobin
HAEMOPTYSIS – Coughing up blood
HAEMOSTASIS – Clotting of the blood
HALITOSIS – Bad breath
HEMICRANIA – Headache affecting one side of the head
HEMIPARESIS – Weakness of one half of the body
HEMIPLEGIA – Paralysis of one half of the body
HEPATOMEGALY – Enlargement of the liver
Hetero- – Different
HISTOLOGY – The study of tissues
Homo- – Same
HORDEOLUM – Stye
HYDROCOELE – Collection of fluid in the scrotum
Hyper- – Excessive
Hypo- – Under, insufficient
HYPOCHONDRIUM – Area of the abdomen beneath the ribs

IATROGENIC – Doctor induced
ICHOR* – Thin, watery discharge from an ulcer
ICTERUS – Jaundice
IDIOPATHIC – Of unknown origin

INCUBUS* – Nightmare
INDURATED – Hardened
INFARCT – Death of part or whole of an organ from lack of blood
Inter- – Between
INTERTRIGO – Rash occurring between two surfaces in contact
ISCHAEMIA – Insufficient blood supply to maintain full function
Iso- – Same
-itis – Suffix applied to organ or tissue indicating inflammation

JACTITION* – Extreme restlessness
JAUNDICE – Excess bile in the blood

KERATITIS – Inflammation of the cornea
KERNICTERUS – Bile deposits in the basal ganglia
KETONURIA – Ketones in the urine
KOILONYCHIA – Spoon-shaped nails
KYPHOSIS – Hunch-backed

LAPAROTOMY – Operation involving opening the abdominal cavity
LAPAROSCOPY – Inspection of the inside of the abdomen
LESION – Local pathological change in a tissue
Leuco- – White
LEUCOCYTOSIS – Increased quantity of leucocytes in the blood
LEUCOPENIA – Decreased quantity of leucocytes in the blood
LIENTERIC* – Presence of fatty stools
LIPOMA – Benign tumour of fatty tissue
LUMEN – Hollow inside of an organ or tube
LYMPHOMA – Tumour of lymphatic tissue
LYSIS – Dissolution

Macro- – Large
MACULE – Flat skin lesion, i.e. a rash
MARASMUS – Severe wasting of baby, 'failure to thrive'
MEATUS – Canal, opening
MELAENA – Passage of dark, digested blood in the stools
MENTAGRA* – Barber's itch
METASTASIS – Spread of disease from one part of body to another
MICTURITION – Urination
Micro- – Small
MILIARY – Wide dissemination resembling millet seeds
MORPHOLOGY – Shape

237

MURAL – Pertaining to a wall or surface
MUSCAE (VOLITANTES) – Floaters in the eye
MYDRIATIC – A drug which dilates the pupil
MYELOID – Pertaining to the bone marrow or spinal cord
Myo- – Muscle
MYOPIC – Short sighted
MYOSITIS – Inflammation of a muscle
MYOTIC – A drug which constricts the pupil

NAEVUS – Benign tumour of blood vessels in skin
NATES* – Buttocks
NECROSIS – Death of tissue
NEOPLASM – Abnormal new growth in a tissue or organ
NEURALGIA – Pain in the distribution of a nerve
NEURASTHENIA* – General weakness
NYSTAGMUS – Involuntary rapid tremor of the eyeballs

OEDEMA – Leakage of fluid into tissues
OLIGO – Insufficient, a few
OLIGURIA – Passing very small quantities of urine
OMENTUM – Fatty tissue in abdominal cavity
ONANISM* – Masturbation
OOPHORITIS – Inflammation of the ovary
OPISTHOTONOUS – Arching of the back
ORCHITIS – Inflammation of the testis
Ortho- – Proper, upright
ORTHOPNOEA – Unable to breath easily when lying flat
-osis – State, condition
OTALGIA – Pain in the ear
OTORRHOEA – Discharge from the ear
-ostomy – Making an opening
-otomy – Cutting, dividing
OZAENA* – Discharging nasal ulcer

PAPILLOEDEMA – Oedema of the optic disc
PAPULE – Raised skin lesion
PARAPLEGIA – Paralysis of both legs
PARONYCHIA – Inflammation of nail bed, whitlow
PAROXYSM – Explosive symptom
PEDUNCULATED – Having a stalk
PERINAEUM – Area between the legs

PERNIO* – Chilblain
PES – Foot
PETECHIAE – Small bruises or haemorrhages in skin
PHAGODENIC* – Flesh-eating ulcer
PHIMOSIS – Tight foreskin
PHTHISIS – Tuberculosis
PLEURODYNIA – Painful intercostal muscles
PLEXUS – A network
Poly- – Many
PRESBYACUSIS – Deafness of advancing age
PRESBYOPIA – Longsightedness of advancing age
PRIAPISM – Painful, involuntary, sustained erection
PROCTITIS – Inflammation of the rectum
PRODROMAL – Transient symptoms preceding the main illness
PURPURA – Rash characterised by widespread bruises
PUSTULE – Small collection of pus under the skin
PYELITIS – Infection of the kidney pelvis
PYREXIA – Fever
PYROSIS* – Heartburn

RALES – Wheezing sound heard in the chest
Retro- – Behind
RIGOR – Severe shivering
RUPIA* – Blistering and scabbing of the skin

SCIRRHUS – Type of carcinoma characterised by hardness
SCLEROSIS – Hardening
SPLENOMEGALY – Enlargement of spleen
SERPIGINOUS – Irregularity (of ulcer)
SINGULTUS* – Hiccup
SORDES – Crusts
SPONDYLOSIS – Condition involving the vertebrae
STEATORRHOEA – Fatty, undigested stools
STENOSIS – Narrowing
STOMA – Aperture, mouth
STRABISMUS – Squint
SUPPURATE – To form pus
SYNCOPE – Fainting
SYNDROME – Collection of symptoms
SYNOVITIS – Inflammation of synovial membrane of joints
SYSTOLE – Contraction phase of the heart

Tachy- – Rapid
TACHYCARDIA – Rapid heart beat
TENESMUS – Painful, ineffectual attempt to empty bowel
TENOSYNOVITIS – Inflammation of tendon sheath
THROMBOSIS – Blood clot
TINNITUS – Ringing in the ears
TORTICOLLIS – Spasm of sternomastoid muscle causing stiff neck

ULCER – Defect in epithelim where tissue is lost
URAEMIA – Presence of excess urea in the blood
URTICARIA – Nettle-rash
UVEA – Area of eye which includes choroid, iris and ciliary body

VARICES – Tortuous, dilated veins
VESICLE – Small blister on skin
VISCERA – Internal organs
VOLVULUS – Blockage of the bowel caused by twisting

WEAL – Raised, itchy lesion in skin
WHITLOW – Infection of the nail bed

APPENDIX
OF USEFUL
ADDRESSES

Lupus Group, Arthritis Care
6 Grosvenor Cres
London SW1X 7ER

Action Against Allergy
43 The Downs
London SW20 8MG

Terence Higgins Trust
54 Graves End Road
London W12

National Osteoporosis Society
Barton Mead House
PO Box 10
Radstock, Bath BA3 3YB

Back Pain Association
Grundy House
31–33 Park Road
Teddington, Middx

Cystic Fibrosis Research Trust
5 Blyth Road, Bromley, Kent

Colostomy Welfare Group
38–39 Eccleston Sq.
London SW1

British Kidney Patient Association
Oakhanger Place, Bordon, Hants

British Diabetic Association
10 Queen Anne St
London W1M 0BD

MS Society of UK
25 Effie Rd
London SW6

MS Society
286 Munster Road
London SW6

UK ME Society
The Moss
Third Ave
Stanford-Le-Hope
Essex SS17 8EL

Parkinson's Disease Society
81 Queen's Road
London SW19

Association for Spina Bifida
Tavistock House North
Tavistock Sq.
London W21

RNIB
224 Portland St
London W1

RNID
(Royal National Institute for the Deaf)
105 Gower Street
London WC1

British Tinnitus Association
Address as for RNID

INDEX